# MATHS SKILLS
# FOR PHARMACY

# MATHS SKILLS FOR PHARMACY

## Unlocking pharmaceutical calculations

Chris **Langley** and Yvonne **Perrie**

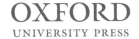
OXFORD
UNIVERSITY PRESS

# OXFORD
UNIVERSITY PRESS

Great Clarendon Street, Oxford, OX2 6DP,
United Kingdom

Oxford University Press is a department of the University of Oxford.
It furthers the University's objective of excellence in research, scholarship,
and education by publishing worldwide. Oxford is a registered trade mark of
Oxford University Press in the UK and in certain other countries

© Chris Langley and Yvonne Perrie 2015

The moral rights of the authors have been asserted

Impression: 8

Published in the United States of America by Oxford University Press
198 Madison Avenue, New York, NY 10016, United States of America

British Library Cataloguing in Publication Data
Data available

Library of Congress Control Number: 2014948247

ISBN 978-0-19-968071-9

Printed in Great Britain by Ashford Colour Press Ltd, Gosport, Hampshire

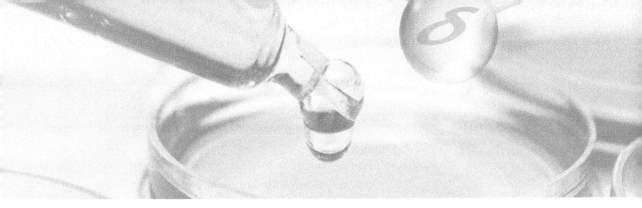

# Preface

It is a fundamental part of the education of student pharmacists and pharmacy technicians that they are able to understand and demonstrate competence in undertaking calculations relating to the correct efficacious supply of medicinal products. Pharmacy students encounter dosage calculations at all stages of their undergraduate studies, and then again within their pre-registration year and onwards into their careers as qualified pharmacists. Therefore, it is imperative that students are supported through this compulsory part of the curricula. To help students achieve this aim, this text has been designed as a core resource for all undergraduate MPharm programmes within the United Kingdom and beyond. In addition, this text will be of use to student pharmacy technicians on their educational journey to registration.

*Maths Skills for Pharmacy* will cover all aspects relating to the calculations encountered in pharmaceutical practice, and also provide support for the calculations behind the dosage forms. Written by two academic pharmacists, this text uniquely brings together mathematical concepts from both the scientific and practice sides of pharmacy to enable pharmacy students and student pharmacy technicians to understand and integrate their knowledge on pharmaceutical calculations.

Christopher A Langley
Yvonne Perrie
July 2014

# How to use this book

*Maths Skills for Pharmacy* features a range of learning features to help you master pharmaceutical calculations and use them in a variety of situations.

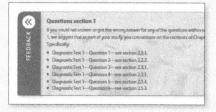

**Diagnostic calculations tests** in Chapter 1 are specifically designed to help you focus your learning. Complete the first diagnostic test and check the answers at the end of Chapter 1 to identify those areas you find the most difficult. Feedback boxes within the answers signpost the specific chapters and sections that you should concentrate on to help you gain confidence in the topics you particularly struggled with. The second of the diagniostic tests is designed to be used following your study of the different chapters to check your understanding and to highlight areas you may wish to focus on again.

**Running case studies** appear throughout the text, featuring a group of patients who are introduced in Chapter 1. These case studies are designed to help you choose the information to include in a calculation when presented with a range of different data about a patient, some of which will not be relevant for the particular calculation(s) in question. Furthermore, they are written to help you develop a patient focus to your studies and understand why maths is such an important part of pharmacy practice.

**Worked examples** throughout every chapter in the book show all the steps you need to undertake in order to reach the final solution to a given question.

**Self-assessment questions** enable you to test your understanding of the topics you have just studied. Answers can be found at the end of each chapter.

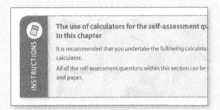

| QUESTION 2.1: | What is 0.45 g in milligrams, micrograms, and nanograms? |
| QUESTION 2.2: | What is 0.578 g in nanograms? |
| QUESTION 2.3: | What is 2345 nanograms in micrograms and milligrams? |
| QUESTION 2.4: | What is 0.75 L in millilitres, microlitres, and nanolitres? |
| QUESTION 2.5: | What is 0.96 L in nanolitres? |
| QUESTION 2.6: | What is 1500 nanolitres in microlitres and millilitres? |
| QUESTION 2.7: | A cream contains 3.5% w/w of active ingredient. How much active ingredient would be present in 150 g of cream? |
| QUESTION 2.8: | A cream contains 15% w/w of active ingredient. How much active ingredient would be present in 500 g of cream? |

**Calculator boxes** explain whether or not a calculator should be used for the questions in that particular chapter or section.

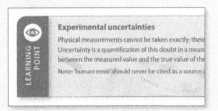

INSTRUCTIONS

**The use of calculators for the self-assessment questions in this chapter**

It is recommended that you undertake the following calculations with a calculator.

All of the self-assessment questions within this section can be [done with] and paper.

**Learning point boxes** highlight the key take-home points to remember having studied each section of a given chapter.

LEARNING POINT

**Experimental uncertainties**

Physical measurements cannot be taken exactly; there [is...] Uncertainty is a quantification of this doubt in a measurement between the measured value and the true value of the [...]

Note: 'human error' should never be cited as a source [...]

# Online Resource Centre

The Online Resource Centre to accompany *Maths Skills for Pharmacy* provides additional teaching and learning resources for students and lecturers.

The site can be accessed at: **www.oxfordtextbooks.co.uk/orc/langley/**

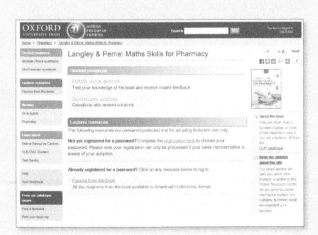

The most effective way to increase your confidence and proficiency with pharmaceutical calculations is to practise the mathematics involved. With this in mind, the online resources provided for students include interactive multiple-choice questions with feedback directing you to specific sections of the book for more information, and short-answer questions with worked solutions.

For registered adopters of the book, figures from the book can be downloaded for use in lecture slides.

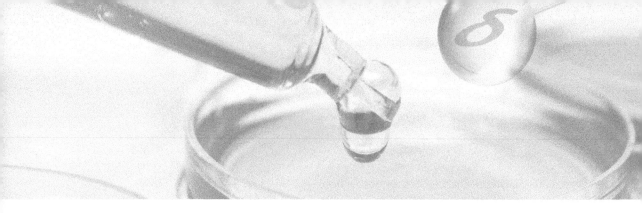

# About the authors

### Professor Chris Langley

**Professor Chris Langley** is Professor of Pharmacy Law and Practice at Aston Pharmacy School, where he specializes in teaching the legal, ethical, and practice components of the undergraduate degree course. In addition, he is currently the Associate Dean for Taught Programmes for the School of Life and Health Sciences within Aston University. His research interests centre on the role of the pharmacist in both primary and secondary care and work examining pharmacy educational policy. Nationally, Chris is a member of the General Pharmaceutical Council's Pre-Registration Board of Assessors, Accreditation and Recognition Panel and the statutory Fitness to Practise Committee. He is also a member of the Royal Pharmaceutical Society's Education Expert Advisory Panel and a Principal Fellow of the Higher Education Academy.

### Professor Yvonne Perrie

**Professor Yvonne Perrie** is the Head of Pharmacy and Chair in Drug Delivery within Aston University. She has a BSc (First-Class Hons) in Pharmacy from Strathclyde University, and a PhD from the University of London under the supervision of Professor Gregoriadis. Yvonne's research is multi-disciplinary and focused on the development of drug carrier systems for the delivery of drugs and vaccines. Yvonne is a Director-at-Large for the Controlled Release Society. She is Editor-in-Chief of the *Journal of Liposome Research and Pharmaceutics* and Associate Editor for the *Journal of Drug Targeting* and the *Journal of Pharmacy and Pharmacology*.

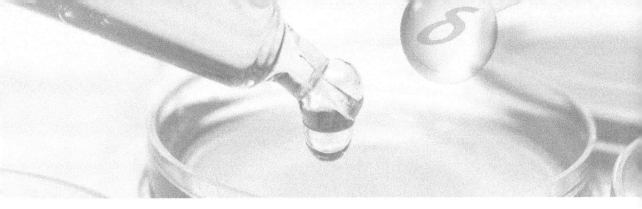

# Contents

# Introduction: the importance of maths in pharmacy

# 1

## 1.1 Introduction to mathematics within healthcare

Whatever sector of the profession a pharmacist or pharmacy technician works within, a fundamental part of any role is the ability to calculate safe and efficacious drug doses. Pharmacists and pharmacy technicians are both vital contributors to the wide multi-disciplinary healthcare team and, as such, must be able to carry out their roles effectively and safely. The importance of being able to calculate accurately dosages of differing drugs for different patients cannot be underestimated. If this role is performed inaccurately or without due care, there is the possibility of the drug not having its desired outcome. This, at best, would cause inconvenience to the patient; however, at worst, it could lead to the patient being seriously harmed or even dying.

For many patients, modern healthcare is a complex interplay between many different healthcare interventions. For example, a patient who has diabetes will be managed with a range of drugs along with other interventions such as diet management and exercise. Here, the medication prescribed forms a core part of the management of the patient's condition. Other healthcare interventions may not primarily focus on the use of drugs; however, drugs may be used to manage symptoms from either the condition or the intervention. For example, a patient with a broken arm will need some form of surgery for the bone to be reset. During this procedure, various drugs would be used; for example, pre-operative medication, anaesthetics during the procedure, and medication to prevent blood clotting. Following the procedure, a range of analgesic and antibiotic medication may also be administered. This means that although the primary intervention was non-pharmacotherapeutic (i.e. the surgery), medication formed an important part of the process before, during, and after the main intervention. Therefore, although there are many healthcare interventions that do not involve the administration of drugs (e.g. management of a patient's weight using advice on diet and exercise), many do use drugs as either a primary or secondary part of the process.

With so many healthcare interventions requiring the administration of some form of medication, it can be seen that the possibility of error is great. Even at very high accuracy levels, with the sheer number of drug doses being prescribed every day, errors are bound to occur. It is the role of the pharmacist and pharmacy technician to ensure that the level of error is kept as low as possible, especially when dealing with certain 'Red Flag' drugs where errors are more likely to result in severe harm to the patient.

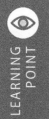

**LEARNING POINT**

### 'Red Flag' drugs

A 'Red Flag' drug is one where additional caution is needed during either the prescribing or supply of the medicine. This may be because of a particular safety issue and/or linked to the likelihood of severe harm if an error is made.

For example, certain does of methotrexate are to be taken once a week. This would be classified as a 'Red Flag' drug as the potential to prescribe or label the medication as a once-daily administration would be high (very few drugs are taken once a week and so it would be quite easy to default to a once-daily dosing by mistake), leading to patient harm.

So where can medication errors occur? Essentially, there are three core places where medication error can take place and all of these can be caused (among other causes) by inaccurate calculations:

- **Prescribing**: Firstly, following the successful diagnosis of a condition, if appropriate, the prescriber will prescribe a dose of a particular drug or drugs. It is at this point that the first error could occur. Many drug doses are straightforward and are therefore less likely to be inaccurate. For example, an adult dose of paracetamol tablets to treat mild to moderate pain in an otherwise healthy individual would be, one to two 500 mg tablets every 4-6 hours, with no more than eight tablets to be taken in any 24-hour period. This dose remains constant for all similar (i.e. otherwise healthy) adults and is not dependent on other patient factors (e.g. the patient's body weight). Conversely, the dose of a reconstituted chemotherapeutic agent for intravenous infusion to treat cancer would vary patient by patient and is based on the patient's body surface area. Therefore, the possibility of calculating an inaccurate dose for patients taking a medication where there is greater inter-patient variability in the dose is much higher as, in this example, the prescriber has first to calculate the patient's body surface area using other information (the patient's height and weight) and then use this information to calculate an accurate dose.

Therefore, it is a core part of the medication supply process that doses of all medication are checked by the supplying pharmacist or pharmacy technician, with any final clinical check forming part of the pharmacist's role. For some drugs, this is a relatively straightforward process but for others additional information may be required such as:

- The *patient's diagnosis*—as the dose of a particular drug can vary dependent on the disease state being treated.
- *Specific patient factors* that may influence the correct dose to be prescribed—such as the patient's weight (as discussed previously).
- *Other drugs* that the patient may be taking—as other drugs may interact with the drug being supplied and result in the need to increase or decrease the dose of one or other drug.

- **Supply**: Secondly, assuming that the dosage has been calculated correctly (as detailed in the previous stage), the pharmacist or pharmacy technician needs to supply the correct medication. Again, in many cases, from a mathematical perspective, this is relatively straightforward; but for the supply of some medication this may be more complex. Using the example from above, if the prescription had called for 100 paracetamol 500 mg tablets, working out the number to be supplied is simple. So long as the correct item is taken from stock, supplying 100 tablets is not, from a mathematical perspective, a difficult task. However, for the example involving the chemotherapy, this would require the calculation of the amount of drug to be reconstituted within a vial and the calculation of the amount of this reconstituted drug to be administered over a particular time frame to the patient.

  The role of pharmacy has expanded over the last 10-20 years, with both pharmacists and pharmacy technicians becoming increasingly involved in a wider range of healthcare activities. Nevertheless, the supply of safe and efficacious medication still remains a core function of the pharmacy profession and, therefore, it is imperative that this task is performed to a high level of accuracy.

- **Administration**: Finally, assuming that the correct medication was prescribed and subsequently supplied (as detailed in the two previous stages), errors are still possible during the administration part of the supply. In order for the medication to be effective, it needs to be administered to the patient either by the patient themself, by someone acting in a caring capacity (e.g. in a residential home for elderly or disabled patients), relatives or parents of the patient, or by healthcare staff (e.g. a nurse on a hospital ward). As in the previous stages, depending on the medication to be taken or administered, this stage of the process may be a relatively straightforward task (e.g. administration of two tablets), through to a task requiring some manipulation of the medication (e.g. administration of 1.25 mL using a suitably graduated oral syringe).

  To minimize the potential for error at the administration stage, it is vital that you are able to understand the differing medication administration techniques and are also able to explain confidently and clearly how to use different medication administration devices to patients, other individuals who may administer medication to patients (e.g. parents), and other healthcare professionals (e.g. ward nursing staff).

With an accurate understanding of the different mathematical manipulations required at each of the three stages outlined above, you will be able to ensure that accurate, safe, and efficacious doses are provided to patients to maximize the benefit provided by their medicines.

---

### Medication errors

Medication errors occur at one or more of three points in the medication administration process, and so it is important that care is taken at all three stages. These stages are the

- *prescribing,*
- *supply,* and
- *administration*

of the drug or drugs for each patient.

LEARNING POINT

# 1.2 The layout of this text

## 1.2.1 Chapter contents

This text has been set out in a number of distinct chapters to reflect the differing types of calculations involved in preparation of safe and efficacious pharmaceutical products. In summary, these chapters are:

### Chapter 1: Introduction: the importance of maths in pharmacy

This chapter sets the scene for the book and outlines the importance of accuracy in pharmaceutical calculations. Concepts around estimation and mechanisms for self-check are discussed, and this is followed by a diagnostic test to allow you to evaluate your own calculations ability. In addition, a summary of the following chapters is provided, along with a brief contextualization of pharmacy calculations in relation to patient care. The key sections within this chapter are:

- Introduction to mathematics within healthcare.
- The layout of this text.
- Getting it right: estimation and self-checking.
- Diagnostic calculations test 1.
- Running case studies: meet the patients.
- Diagnostic calculations test 2.

### Chapter 2: Pharmaceutical mathematical terminology

This chapter outlines and explains in detail all the key terminology relating to pharmaceutical calculations. In addition, this chapter explains conversion of major units between imperial and metric systems. Each different pharmaceutical term is introduced and then its use explained by the employment of suitable practice-based examples. A series of self-assessment questions (including running case studies) will then follow to allow you to self-evaluate your own learning. The key sections within this chapter are:

- Chapter introduction.
- Converting between standard units.
- Specific pharmaceutical mathematical terminology.
- Interpreting dosage instructions.
- Imperial and metric conversions.
- Self-assessment questions (including running case studies).
- Summary.
- Answers to self-assessment questions.

### Chapter 3: Mathematical basics in pharmacy: measurements and data

Building on preceding material, this chapter changes focus and discusses the basics of the mathematics relating to pharmaceutical sciences. Concentrating on the basics first, and using a range of worked examples, a range of concepts are covered including experimental uncertainties, data averages, data variability, and accuracy and precision. The key sections within this chapter are:

- Chapter introduction.
- Variation in measurements and experimental uncertainties.
- Accuracy and precision.

- Data sets: samples and populations.
- Calculating the average of data sets.
- Measurement of the variability of data.
- Self-assessment questions (including running case studies).
- Summary.
- Answers to self-assessment questions.

## Chapter 4: Maths supporting the science of pharmacy

This chapter continues with examination of calculations relating to the core pharmaceutical sciences by discussing the following: displacement, freezing points, molarity, and molecular concentration. As with other chapters, worked examples and student self-assessment questions are employed to assist you in becoming competent with calculations around the presented concepts. The key sections within this chapter are:

- Chapter introduction.
- Displacement values and volumes.
- Iso-osmotic and isotonic solutions: considerations for formulations.
- Preparing isotonic solutions.
- Self-assessment questions (including running case studies).
- Summary.
- Answers to self-assessment questions.

## Chapter 5: Quantities to dispense: accuracy within supply

This chapter covers all aspects of pharmaceutical calculations relating to the quantities of medicines to dispense in relation to different medication orders. Aspects of dispensing relating to 'special containers' are covered, as is the supply of medication affected by expiry of the medicinal product during the period of supply (e.g. the supply of paediatric antibiotic suspensions). The key sections within this chapter are:

- Chapter introduction.
- Basic quantity calculations: solid dosage forms.
- Basic quantity calculations: liquid dosage forms.
- Basic quantity calculations: special containers.
- Quantity calculations: intravenous infusions.
- Expiration of medication during the supply period.
- Self-assessment questions (including running case studies).
- Summary.
- Answers to self-assessment questions.

## Chapter 6: Handling pharmaceutical products: concentrations and dilutions

The ability of a pharmacist and pharmacy technician to undertake accurate calculations relating to concentrations and dilutions of pharmaceutical preparations is a key part of good pharmaceutical practice. This core chapter sets out, in a number of defined sections, to assist you in understanding the various mathematical manipulations involved. The key sections within this chapter are:

- Chapter introduction.
- Percentages and ratios.

- Preparing concentrated solutions.
- Diluting solutions.
- Alligation.
- Self-assessment questions (including running case studies).
- Summary.
- Answers to self-assessment questions.

### Chapter 7: Intravenous and associated medication routes

Following on from Chapter 6, this chapter discusses the mathematics involved in calculating the appropriate administration rate, principally for intravenous medication. Furthermore, conversion between oral and intravenous administration rates (e.g. for morphine) is also covered. The key sections within this chapter are:

- Chapter introduction.
- Basic intravenous infusion rates.
- Variable intravenous infusion rates.
- Converting oral administration rates to other routes.
- Infusion administration methods.
- Self-assessment questions (including running case studies).
- Summary.
- Answers to self-assessment questions.

### Chapter 8: Data: presentation, interpretation, and basic statistics

In addition to calculations relating to patient-facing dosage forms, it is necessary that pharmacists and pharmacy technicians understand the concepts of data presentation and basic statistics to allow for successful integration with the pharmaceutical sciences. The key sections within this chapter are:

- Chapter introduction.
- Presentation of data using tables and graphs.
- Linear and logarithmic calculations.
- Stability of medicines.
- Simple statistics: analysis of data.
- Self-assessment questions (including running case studies).
- Summary.
- Answers to self-assessment questions.

### Appendix: Pharmaceutical administration abbreviations

Following the main chapters of the text, an appendix is provided that lists all the main Latin abbreviations commonly used to indicate administration instructions on prescriptions.

### 1.2.2 Running case studies

Throughout this text, in addition to the basic self-assessment questions found towards the end of each chapter, there will be a series of running case studies. These sets of questions will be based around the same set of patients (who are introduced in section 1.5) and, in addition to performing the correct mathematical calculation, you will be required to 'extract' the correct patient-specific factors from the patients' profiles as required. When undertaking calculations relating to drug dosages in a real-life clinical setting, more often than not, when it is necessary to obtain specific patient information, it is necessary to extract this information from, for example, patient notes. Therefore, these questions have been designed in this way to mimic real-life scenarios more realistically.

# 1.3 Getting it right: estimation and self-checking

## 1.3.1 Estimation

As outlined in the previous section, it is important that all calculations relating to the prescribing, supply, and administration of pharmacotherapeutic dosage forms are accurate. In a real clinical setting, many of these calculations will be performed and/or checked using a calculator. This is done for a number of reasons, one of the primary ones being that the figures used do not often lend themselves to easy calculation using a pen and paper, and, in theory (i.e. so long as the correct figures are entered into the calculator), unlike a human, the calculator won't make simple arithmetic mistakes.

However, the danger of simple reliance on a calculator is that it is easy to believe what the calculator is showing us. Put the wrong figures into a calculator and you will get the wrong answer out. To tackle this issue, many courses undertaken pre-qualification (e.g. the MPharm pharmacy degree course) have a medication calculations component that does not permit the use of calculators. For this to work, often the calculation questions are 'cleansed', that is they have been deliberately written so as to be relatively straightforward to calculate without the use of a calculator (e.g. in many cases, steps involving values with many decimal places have been avoided). In addition to helping you practise basic arithmetic calculations, what this also does is help you to develop an ability to estimate the magnitude of an answer. This, in turn, helps you to identify incorrect answers more easily by having a 'feel' for what the right answer should be.

| | **EXAMPLE 1:1** |
|---|---|
| **Question:** | You are asked to calculate the amount of Ingredient A in 25 g of a cream, where there are 45 g of Ingredient A in 100 g of the cream. |
| **Answer:** | Before you even attempt the calculation, you should be estimating the mathematical range the answer would lie within. If there are 45 g of Ingredient A in 100 g of the cream, the amount of Ingredient A is just below half of the total amount. Therefore, the amount of Ingredient A in 25 g of the cream should be just below half of 25 g, that is somewhere below, but not too far away from, 12.5 g. |
| | Then attempt the calculation. If there are 45 g of Ingredient A in 100 g of the cream, in 25 g there are: |
| | $$(45 \div 100) \times 25 = 11.25 \, g.$$ |
| | Therefore, there would be 11.25 g of Ingredient A in 25 g of the cream. This, you will note, is somewhere below, but not too far away from 12.5 g. |

| | EXAMPLE 1:2 |
|---|---|
| **Question:** | A patient requires a dose of Drug B at 20 mg/m². The patient has a body surface area of 1.8 m². |
| **Answer:** | Before you even attempt the calculation, you should be estimating the mathematical range the answer would be within. In this case, the dose of Drug B would be 20 mg for every square metre of body surface area. As the patient's body surface area is below, but not too far from 2 m², we would expect the answer to be less than, but not too far from 40 mg (i.e. 20 mg × 2). |
| | Then attempt the calculation. If every square metre of body surface area requires a dose of 20 mg, for a patient with a body surface area of 1.8 m², the dose would be: |
| | $$20 \times 1.8 = 36\,\text{mg}.$$ |
| | Therefore, the patient requires a dose of 36 mg. This, you will note, is somewhere below, but not too far away from 40 mg. |

In both these examples, you can see how estimation of the answer provided confirmation that the calculated value was of the right magnitude. Had, for example, the calculated answer for Example 1:1 been inaccurately calculated as 13.5 g, it would have been easy to see that this is incorrect as it is above (rather than being just below) 12.5 g. Therefore, by developing an ability to estimate the magnitude of the answer from a dosage calculation, you are easily able to self-check answers and potentially identify errors.

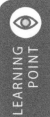

### Estimation

If you are able to estimate the answer to a pharmaceutical calculation, you can use this estimated answer to check the likelihood that the final calculated answer is correct. If there is a big difference between the estimated answer and the calculated answer, it is worth double-checking any calculations.

LEARNING POINT

### 1.3.2 Self-checking

In addition to estimation, which is used to gauge the likelihood that an answer produced in response to a particular pharmaceutical dosage query is correct, it is also important that you develop the ability to self-check answers. There are essentially three primary ways to achieve this.

Firstly, you can simply repeat the calculation and see if the same answer is obtained. The advantage of this method is that it is relatively straightforward to undertake (as, if you were able to perform the calculation once, from a mathematical perspective, repeating the calculations should be relatively straightforward). However, linked to this point, the main disadvantage of this method is that if a calculation manipulation error was made in the primary calculation, then it is likely that the error would occur again in the secondary (checking) calculation.

| | **EXAMPLE 1:3** |
|---|---|
| **Question:** | A patient requires a dose of Drug C at 15 mg/m². The patient has a body surface area of 1.9 m². |
| **Answer:** | Before you even attempt the calculation, you should be estimating the mathematical range the answer would be within. In this case, the dose of Drug C would be 15 mg for every square metre of body surface area. As the patient's body surface area is below, but not too far from 2 m², we would expect the answer to be less than, but not too far from 30 mg (i.e. 15 mg×2). |
| | If every square metre of body surface area requires a dose of 15 mg, for a patient with a body surface area of 1.9 m², the dose would be: |
| | $15 \times 1.9 = 28.5$ mg. |
| | However, if an error is made in the calculation of the answer, an incorrect dose of, for example, 27.5 mg could be calculated. |
| | As you will see from the figures above, simply relying on an estimation of the scale of the correct answer does not immediately indicate that the calculated dosage value is incorrect (i.e. the difference between the correct value of 28.5 mg and the incorrect value of 27.5 mg is not instantly noticeable as both are slightly below our estimated value of 30 mg). |
| | Therefore, in addition to estimating the magnitude of the answer, we also need to check the value we have obtained. However, although it is relatively straightforward to calculate a second answer using the same methodology, in checking this calculation using the method where the calculation is repeated, the danger is that the initial calculation error would not be noticed and the erroneous answer 27.5 mg also be repeated. As the estimation of the magnitude of the answer has not indicated any problem with the answer, this value, having been calculated twice, is likely to be erroneously accepted as being correct. |

The second method of checking an answer is correct is to repeat the calculation but to use an alternative method to the one originally used. To understand this, we need to examine the methodology used for the individual multiplication calculation.

| | **EXAMPLE 1:4** |
|---|---|
| **Question:** | A patient requires a dose of Drug C at 15 mg/m². The patient has a body surface area of 1.9 m². |
| **Answer:** | Before you even attempt the calculation, you should be estimating the mathematical range the answer would be within. In this case, the dose of Drug C would be 15 mg for every square metre of body surface area. As the patient's body surface area is below, but not too far from 2 m², we would expect the answer to be less than, but not too far from 30 mg (i.e. 15 mg×2). |
| | If every square metre of body surface area requires a dose of 15 mg, for a patient with a body surface area of 1.9 m², the dose would be: |
| | $15 \times 1.9 = 28.5$ mg. |

To calculate this answer, the following methodology was used to obtain the answer:

Firstly, remove the decimal:

$$15 \times 1.9 \equiv (15 \times 19) \div 10.$$

Then, using a standard multiplication technique, multiply the two figures within the brackets.

$$15 \times 19 = 285.$$

Then divide this figure by 10 to give the final answer:

$$285 \div 10 = 28.5 \, \text{mg}.$$

To check this answer, undertake the calculation a different way:

In this example, we need to multiply 15 by a number just less than 2. Therefore, it would be fairly straightforward to calculate the answer an alternative way by taking 2 multiplied by 15 and then subtracting from that value 0.1 multiplied by 15, i.e.:

$$15 \times 1.9 \equiv (15 \times 2) - (15 \times 0.1).$$

This is equivalent to:

$$30 - (15 \times 0.1) \equiv 30 - 1.5 = 28.5 \, \text{mg}.$$

Therefore, we have used a different way to calculate the dosage but have come to the same answer. This indicates that it is more likely to be correct than simply calculating the answer using the same methodology twice.

The third method we can use to check an answer is to use the answer in a further calculation. This method differs slightly to the previous two methods as, unlike the first two, we are using the answer to check the calculation, rather than simply repeating the calculation by either using the same or a different calculation methodology.

| EXAMPLE 1:5 | |
|---|---|
| **Question:** | A patient requires a dose of Drug C at 15 mg/m². The patient has a body surface area of 1.9 m². |
| **Answer:** | Before you even attempt the calculation, you should be estimating the mathematical range the answer would be within. In this case, the dose of Drug C would be 15 mg for every square metre of body surface area. As the patient's body surface area is below, but not too far from 2 m², we would expect the answer to be less than, but not too far from 30 mg (i.e. 15 mg × 2). |
| | If every square metre of body surface area requires a dose of 15 mg, for a patient with a body surface area of 1.9 m², the dose would be: |
| | $$15 \times 1.9 = 28.5 \, \text{mg}.$$ |
| | To check this answer, we can take the answer we have calculated (28.5 mg) and use it to calculate one of the original values. This is the equivalent of saying either: |
| | a) For a dose of 28.5 mg and a prescribed dose of 15 mg/m², what is the body surface area of the patient? |

Or

    b) For a dose of 28.5 mg and a body surface area of 1.9 m², what is the prescribed dose of the medication?

If we calculate the answer to (a) and/or (b) above and obtain the answer(s) 1.9 m² and/or 15 mg/m², we can be more confident that the originally calculated answer of 28.5 mg is correct.

If the dose is 28.5 mg and the patient has been prescribed a dose of 15 mg/m², then the body surface area of the patient is:

$$28.5 \div 15 = 1.9 \, m^2.$$

If the dose is 28.5 mg and the body surface area is 1.9 m², then the prescribed dose of the medication is:

$$28.5 \div 1.9 = 15 \, mg/m^2.$$

As either (or both, if both of the calculations were employed) of these calculations have produced the correct value from the original question, we can be more confident that the original answer is correct.

**Self-checking**

LEARNING POINT

Although estimation is a useful tool to help you check whether an answer is likely to be correct, it is useful to combine this with self-checking. Essentially, there are three ways to self-check:

- *Repeat the calculation*—this is easy to do, but can result in the same mistake happening again.
- *Undertake the calculation a different way*—this will potentially avoid any mistakes simply being repeated, but it may not always be possible to easily undertake a calculation in a different way.
- *Use the answer in a subsequent calculation*—this will potentially avoid any mistakes simply being repeated, but depending on the original calculation, it may not always be possible to undertake a subsequent calculation using the answer obtained.

# 1.4 Diagnostic calculations test 1

This text has been set out in a number of chapters, which have been designed to help you master the differing types of calculations commonly encountered within modern pharmaceutical practice. In essence, most calculations relating to dosages are, once stripped down to the basic figures, simple arithmetic calculations. However, it is useful to group certain types of calculation together to help you to understand how to tackle certain types of calculation and so we have set this text out into different chapters which reflect these groupings. In addition, we are aware that students' abilities to undertake the differing types of calculation (based on these groupings) will vary;

some of you will be comfortable with certain types of calculation and less comfortable with others.

The purpose of the diagnostic calculations test is to enable you to focus on particular areas of the text which cover the material more suited to your own particular calculation needs. Therefore, by undertaking the test in full, you will be guided on the chapters of the text which you may find the most useful. Although we strongly recommend that you familiarize yourself with this text in its entirety, we are aware that some of you will only want to focus on the areas in which you are weakest. This diagnostic calculations test will help you focus your study and/or revision.

### 1.4.1 Diagnostic calculations test

This test has been designed to be undertaken at the beginning of your studies and/ or revision on pharmaceutical calculations. It is recommended that you undertake the whole test in one sitting and only use a calculator for those questions where it is stated that it is permitted. Once you have answered all questions, and checked your answers yourself, you can refer to the answers to the questions at the end of this section (see section 1.4.2). In addition to the answers, this section will also provide guidance on the chapters and/or sections on which to focus should you have found any particular questions difficult.

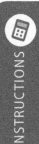

**INSTRUCTIONS**

### The use of calculators during diagnostic calculations test 1

It is recommended that you undertake some of the calculations within this diagnostic calculations test without the use of a calculator.

Unless stated otherwise, all of the self-assessment questions within this test can be undertaken using a pen and paper.

### Diagnostic calculations test 1

#### Section 1

**QUESTION 1:** *What is 0.589 g in milligrams, micrograms, and nanograms?*

**QUESTION 2:** *What is 0.145 L in nanolitres?*

**QUESTION 3:** *A cream contains 0.225% w/w of active ingredient. How much active ingredient would be present in 75 g of cream?*

**QUESTION 4:** *How much active ingredient is present in 250 mL of a 5.5% v/v solution?*

**QUESTION 5:** *How much of a liquid ingredient is required for 1200 mL of a 1 in 15 solution?*

**QUESTION 6:** *A patient has been advised to lose 2.5 kg and wants to know what weight this is in pounds (noting that 2.2 pounds ≈ 1 kg).*

## Diagnostic calculations test 1

### Section 2

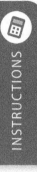

**The use of calculators for the diagnostic assessment questions in section 2**

It is recommended that you undertake the calculations in section 2 using a calculator.

INSTRUCTIONS

**QUESTION 7:** *How many significant figures do the following values contain?*

    *a) 0.00777.*

    *b) 0.03016.*

    *c) 0.031002.*

    *d) 6.39.*

**QUESTION 8:** *A researcher requires 50 mL of water. To measure this, the researcher uses a 10 mL measuring cylinder (which has an associated uncertainty of 0.1 mL) to measure out five lots of 10 mL that are combined to give the researcher a total of 50 mL. Use the range method to estimate the associated uncertainty.*

**QUESTION 9:** *$12.1 \pm 0.1$ g of drug is mixed with $101.6 \pm 0.5$ g of diluent. What is the total weight and the uncertainty of this blend?*

**QUESTION 10:** *A 500 mL infusion bag was prepared to contain 500 mg of drug. Analysis of the contents determined that the infusion bag contained 513 mg of drug. What was the absolute error, the relative error, and percentage relative error associated with this measurement?*

**QUESTION 11:** *The following serum concentrations of fluoxetine were collected:*

*Concentration (nanograms/mL): 220, 260, 240, 255, 240.*

*Calculate the following (assume this is a sample data set):*

    *a) Mean, median, mode.*

    *b) Mean deviation.*

    *c) Variance.*

    *d) Standard deviation.*

    *e) Standard error.*

    *f) % coefficient of variation.*

## Diagnostic calculations test 1
### Section 3

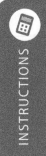

### The use of calculators for the diagnostic assessment questions in section 3.

It is recommended that you undertake the calculations in section 3 using a calculator.

**QUESTION 12:**   *The reconstitution instructions for a dry powder of ampicillin to be prepared as an oral suspension requires the addition of 72 mL of water to give a final volume of 100 mL at a concentration of 125 mg ampicillin in 5 mL. What is the displacement volume for the suspension powder?*

**QUESTION 13:**   *You are asked to prepare six suppositories using 2 g nominal moulds each containing 150 mg of paracetamol and using theobroma oil as the base. The displacement value of paracetamol is 1.5. To allow for wastage, you calculate for eight suppositories. What is the mass of paracetamol and base you require?*

**QUESTION 14:**   *1% w/v of pilocarpine nitrate solution freezes at −0.14°C. What concentration of NaCl (as w/v) is required to make this solution isotonic with blood? What mass of NaCl will be required to prepare a 30 mL solution? Note a 1% w/v of NaCl solution freezes at −0.576°C and an isotonic solution freezes at −0.52°C.*

**QUESTION 15:**   *What is the osmolarity of 0.9% glucose? The molecular weight of glucose is 180 g/mol.*

**QUESTION 16:**   *What mass of NaCl should be added to 50 mL of a 0.5% w/v ammonium chloride solution to make it isotonic with blood (sodium chloride equivalent of ammonium chloride is 1.08)?*

## Diagnostic calculations test 1
### Section 4

**QUESTION 17:**   *You are asked to supply one month's course of medication where the patient has been advised to take one tablet three times a day. How many tablets are required?*

**QUESTION 18:**   *You are asked to supply the following course of prednisolone 5 mg tablets:*

- *4 OD 2/7.*
- *3 OD 2/7.*
- *2 OD 2/7.*
- *1 OD 2/7.*

*How many tablets should you supply?*

**QUESTION 19:** *You are asked to calculate a sufficient quantity (not including an overage) for the following prescription:*

> • *7.5 mL to be taken three times a day for 10 days.*

**QUESTION 20:** *You are asked to supply a sufficient quantity of inhalers (50 inhalations per inhaler) for the following prescription:*

> • *One puff to be inhaled four times a day for 2 months.*

**QUESTION 21:** *You are asked to supply a sufficient quantity of an infusion for the following prescription:*

> • *Prepare a 5 mg/1 mL infusion and administer 400 mg over a 3-hour period.*

## Diagnostic calculations test 1

### Section 5

**QUESTION 22:** *You are asked to make 800 mL pharmaceutical product which contains 2.75% w/v of a drug. How much active ingredient is required?*

**QUESTION 23:** *You are required to make 560 mL of a 1 to 15 solution of a drug (a liquid). How much drug is required?*

**QUESTION 24:** *What is the concentration of a product in percentage which contains a drug in a concentration of 1 in 2.6?*

**QUESTION 25:** *You are required to make 2.6 L of a 1.25% w/v solution of a drug. How much active ingredient is required?*

**QUESTION 26:** *You are required to make 225 mL of an 8% w/v solution of a drug from a 10% solution. How much of the more concentrated solution is required?*

**QUESTION 27:** *You are asked to produce 200 g of a 5% cream using stock creams of 10% and 2%. How much of each stock cream will you require?*

## Diagnostic calculations test 1

### Section 6

**QUESTION 28:** *You are asked to calculate the amount of a drug required to make 125 mL of infusion where the administration rate is 10 mL/min and the dose is 75 mg/min.*

**QUESTION 29:** *You are asked to calculate the infusion rate, in mL/hour, for a 700 mL solution of a drug at a concentration of 50 mg/25 mL and a required dosage of 350 micrograms/min.*

**QUESTION 30:** *Calculate the volume of solution required for an infusion of a drug, at a concentration of 75 mg/5 mL, where you are asked to infuse a total of 1500 mg.*

**QUESTION 31:** *An infusion of a drug is to be delivered at a dose of 5 mg/kg/hour for 6 hours. After this time, the dose is reduced to 3 mg/kg/hour. How long would a 125 mL infusion bag at a concentration of 30 mg/mL last if the patient weighs 70 kg?*

**QUESTION 32:** *A patient requires a dose of 4 mg/hour of a drug. The solution in the syringe is 2 mg/mL and the syringe contains 50 mL and is 10 cm long. At what administration rate, in mm/hour, is the machine required to be set?*

## Diagnostic calculations test 1

### Section 7

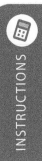

### The use of calculators for the diagnostic assessment questions in section 7.

It is recommended that you undertake the calculations in section 7 using a calculator.

**QUESTION 33:** *Deduce the equation of the straight line given that the gradient of the line is 4.3 and the line passes through the point (8.6,2).*

**QUESTION 34:** *Log linearize the following functions:*

   *a)  $y = 10x^2$.*

   *b)  $y = kx^m$.*

   *c)  $y = km^x$.*

   *d)  $C_t = C_0 \cdot e^{-kt}$.*

**QUESTION 35:** *To investigate the stability of a drug in solution, the drug concentration is measured over time. The degradation process is shown to follow zero order kinetics. If the initial drug concentration is 100 mg/mL, what concentration will be remaining after 5 days if the rate constant $k_0 = 1.60\,day^{-1}$?*

**QUESTION 36:** *In the above example, calculate the overage required to ensure a drug concentration of 95 mg/mL after 6 days.*

**QUESTION 37:** *Consider the following results from a clinical trial. From the table, calculate the standard error of the mean and the 95% confidence interval for both groups and consider if the results are significantly different.*

| | Clinical response Mean (SD) |
| --- | --- |
| **Group A (n=123)** | 77.5 (9.6) |
| **Group B (n=111)** | 61.0 (7.4) |

## 1.4.2  Answers to diagnostic calculations test

This section contains the worked answers for diagnostic calculations test 1.

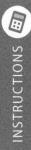

## The use of calculators during diagnostic calculations test 1

It is recommended that you undertake some of the calculations within this diagnostic calculations test without the use of a calculator.

Unless stated otherwise, all of the self-assessment questions within this test can be undertaken using a pen and paper.

## Diagnostic calculations test 1

### Section 1

---

**QUESTION 1:** *What is 0.589 g in milligrams, micrograms, and nanograms?*

**ANSWER:** This calculation involves moving down the weight units in multiples of 1000. Therefore:

> 0.589 g in milligrams = 0.589 × 1000 = 589 mg.

Continuing down the weight units, we can move from milligrams to micrograms by multiplying by another 1000.

> 589 mg (0.589 g) in micrograms = 589 × 1000 = 589 000 micrograms.

Continuing down the weight units, we can move from micrograms to nanograms by multiplying by another 1000.

> 589 000 micrograms (589 mg; 0.589 g) in nanograms
> = 589 000 × 1000 = 589 000 000 nanograms.

---

**QUESTION 2:** *What is 0.145 L in nanolitres?*

**ANSWER:** This calculation involves moving down the volume units in multiples of 1000. However, in this case, the question asks for the answer in nanolitres, without reporting the intermediate units (i.e. the millilitres and the microlitres). Rather than moving straight from litres to nanolitres, it is suggested that you attempt the question in stages, moving through the intermediary units. Therefore:

> 0.145 L in millilitres = 0.145 × 1000 = 145 mL.

Continuing down the volume units, we can move from millilitres to microlitres by multiplying by another 1000.

> 145 mL (0.145 L) in microlitres = 145 × 1000 = 145 000 microlitres.

Continuing down the volume units, we can move from microlitres to nanolitres by multiplying by another 1000.

> 145 000 microlitres (145 mL; 0.145 L) in nanolitres
> = 145 000 × 1000 = 145 000 000 nanolitres.

---

**QUESTION 3:** *A cream contains 0.225% w/w of active ingredient. How much active ingredient would be present in 75 g of cream?*

**ANSWER:** If the cream contains 0.225% w/w of active ingredient, this means that there is 0.225 g in every 100 g of product. Therefore, in 75 g there would be:

$$(0.225 \div 100) \times 75 = 0.16875 \, g = 168.75 \, mg.$$

Therefore, there are 168.75 mg of active ingredient in 75 g of the cream.

**QUESTION 4:** *How much active ingredient is present in 250 mL of a 5.5% v/v solution?*

**ANSWER:** If the final pharmaceutical product contains 5.5% v/v, this means that there are 5.5 mL in every 100 mL of the product. Therefore, in 250 mL of product, there would be:

$$(5.5 \div 100) \times 250 = 13.75 \, mL.$$

Therefore, there are 13.75 mL of active ingredient in 250 mL of the solution.

**QUESTION 5:** *How much of a liquid ingredient is required for 1200 mL of a 1 in 15 solution?*

**ANSWER:** If the solute is to be added to form a 1 in 15 solution, this means that for every 15 mL of solution, 1 mL will be solute. Therefore in 1200 mL, there will be:

$$1200 \div 15 = 80 \, mL \text{ of the liquid ingredient.}$$

Therefore, we require 80 mL of the ingredient (and dissolve this in $(1200 - 80) = 1120 \, mL$ of solvent).

**QUESTION 6:** *A patient has been advised to lose 2.5 kg and wants to know what weight this is in pounds (noting that 2.2 pounds ≈ 1 kg).*

**ANSWER:** For this calculation, we need to multiply the number of kilograms by the conversion factor to obtain the number of pounds the patient has been advised to lose.

$$2.5 \times 2.2 = 5.5 \, lb.$$

Therefore, you need to advise the patient that 2.5 kg is (approximately) the same as 5.5 lb.

FEEDBACK

## Questions section 1

If you could not answer or got the wrong answer for any of the questions within section 1, we suggest that as part of your study, you concentrate on the contents of Chapter 2. Specifically:

- Diagnostic Test 1—Question 1—see section 2.2.1.
- Diagnostic Test 1—Question 2—see section 2.2.2.
- Diagnostic Test 1—Question 3—see section 2.3.1.
- Diagnostic Test 1—Question 4—see section 2.3.1.
- Diagnostic Test 1—Question 5—see section 2.3.4.
- Diagnostic Test 1—Question 6—see section 2.5.3.

## Diagnostic calculations test 1

### Section 2

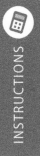

**The use of calculators for the diagnostic assessment questions in section 2**

It is recommended that you undertake the calculations in section 2 using a calculator.

INSTRUCTIONS

---

**QUESTION 7:** *How many significant figures do the following values contain?*

    *a) 0.00777.*

    *b) 0.03016.*

    *c) 0.031002.*

    *d) 6.39.*

**ANSWER:** Count from the first non-zero value:

    a) 0.00777 (3 significant figures).

    b) 0.03016 (4 significant figures).

    c) 0.031002 (5 significant figures).

    d) 6.39 (3 significant figures).

---

**QUESTION 8:** *A researcher requires 50 mL of water. To measure this, the researcher uses a 10 mL measuring cylinder (which has an associated uncertainty of 0.1 mL) to measure out five lots of 10 mL that are combined to give the researcher a total of 50 mL. Use the range method to estimate the associated uncertainty.*

**ANSWER:** 0.5 mL

---

**QUESTION 9:** *12.1±0.1 g of drug is mixed with 101.6±0.5 g of diluent. What is the total weight and the uncertainty of this blend?*

**ANSWER:** 113.7±0.5 g

---

**QUESTION 10:** *A 500 mL infusion bag was prepared to contain 500 mg of drug. Analysis of the contents determined that the infusion bag contained 513 mg of drug. What was the absolute error, the relative error, and percentage relative error associated with this measurement?*

**ANSWER:** The absolute error is 13 mg, the relative error is 0.026, and the percentage relative error is 2.6%.

**QUESTION 11:**   *The following serum concentrations of fluoxetine were collected:*
*Concentration (nanograms/mL): 220, 260, 240, 255, 240.*
*Calculate the following (assume this is a sample data set):*

    a) *Mean, median, mode.*

    b) *Mean deviation.*

    c) *Variance.*

    d) *Standard deviation.*

    e) *Standard error.*

    f) *% coefficient of variation.*

**ANSWER:**   a)   Mean = 243 nanograms/mL, median = 240 nanograms/mL, mode = 240 nanograms/mL.

    b)   Mean deviation = 11.6 nanograms/mL.

    c)   Variance = 245.

    d)   Standard deviation = 15.7 nanograms/mL.

    e)   Standard error = 7.00 nanograms/mL.

    f)   % coefficient of variation = 6.44%.

---

## Questions section 2

**FEEDBACK**

If you could not answer or got the wrong answer for any of the questions within section 2, we suggest that as part of your study, you concentrate on the contents of Chapter 3. Specifically:

- Diagnostic Test 1—Question 7—see section 3.2.1
- Diagnostic Test 1—Question 8—see section 3.2.2.
- Diagnostic Test 1—Question 9—see section 3.2.2.
- Diagnostic Test 1—Question 10—see section 3.3.1.
- Diagnostic Test 1—Question 11—see section 3.5.

## Diagnostic calculations test 1

### Section 3

## The use of calculators for the diagnostic assessment questions in section 3

**INSTRUCTIONS**

It is recommended that you undertake the calculations in section 3 using a calculator.

**QUESTION 12:** *The reconstitution instructions for a dry powder of ampicillin to be prepared as an oral suspension require addition of 72 mL of water to give a final volume of 100 mL at a concentration of 125 mg ampicillin in 5 mL. What is the displacement volume for the suspension powder?*

**ANSWER:** 28 mL/container content.

**QUESTION 13:** *You are asked to prepare six suppositories using 2 g nominal moulds each containing 150 mg of paracetamol and using theobroma oil as the base. The displacement value of paracetamol is 1.5. To allow for wastage, you calculate for eight suppositories. What is the mass of paracetamol and base you require?*

**ANSWER:** Mass of paracetamol = 1200 mg; total amount of base = 15.2 g.

**QUESTION 14:** *1% w/v of pilocarpine nitrate solution freezes at −0.14°C. What concentration of NaCl (as w/v) is required to make this solution isotonic with blood? What mass of NaCl will be required to prepare a 30 mL solution? Note a 1% w/v of NaCl solution freezes at -0.576°C and an isotonic solution freezes at −0.52°C.*

**ANSWER:** 0.66% w/v of NaCl is required. Therefore for 30 mL, 0.20 g of NaCl is required.

**QUESTION 15:** *What is the osmolarity of 0.9% glucose? The molecular weight of glucose is 180 g/mol.*

**ANSWER:** Glucose does not dissociate and has one osmotically active species; therefore the osmolarity of the solution is 0.05 mol/L.

**QUESTION 16:** *What mass of NaCl should be added to 50 mL of a 0.5 % w/v ammonium chloride solution to make it isotonic with blood (sodium chloride equivalent of ammonium chloride is 1.08)?*

**ANSWER:** For 50 mL, 0.18 g NaCl is required.

## Questions section 3

If you could not answer or got the wrong answer for any of the questions within section 3, we suggest that as part of your study, you concentrate on the contents of Chapter 4. Specifically:

- Diagnostic Test 1—Question 12—see section 4.2.1.
- Diagnostic Test 1—Question 13—see section 4.2.2.
- Diagnostic Test 1—Question 14—see section 4.4.1.
- Diagnostic Test 1—Question 15—see section 4.4.2.
- Diagnostic Test 1—Question 16—see section 4.4.4.

FEEDBACK

## Diagnostic calculations test 1

### Section 4

**QUESTION 17:** *You are asked to supply one month's course of medication where the patient has been advised to take one tablet three times a day. How many tablets are required?*

**ANSWER:** In this case, there is no additional information as to the amount of medication to be supplied and so each month can be taken to be 28 days.

For one month's course, we will require:

- $3 \times 28 = 84$ tablets.

Therefore, you need to supply 84 tablets to cover the one-month course of medication.

---

**QUESTION 18:** *You are asked to supply the following course of prednisolone 5 mg tablets:*

- *4 OD 2/7.*
- *3 OD 2/7.*
- *2 OD 2/7.*
- *1 OD 2/7.*

*How many tablets should you supply?*

**ANSWER:** This is a reducing dose of 5 mg prednisolone tablets. The best way to work out the total number of tablets to be supplied is to work it out on a day-by-day basis.

This works out as follows:

- Four daily for 2 days = eight tablets.
- Three daily for 2 days = six tablets.
- Two daily for 2 days = four tablets.
- One daily for 2 days = two tablets.

Therefore the total is 20 tablets.

Therefore, you need to supply 20 tablets to cover the entire reducing course of the 5 mg prednisolone tablets.

---

**QUESTION 19:** *You are asked to calculate a sufficient quantity (not including an overage) for the following prescription:*

- *7.5 mL to be taken three times a day for 10 days.*

**ANSWER:** To work out the total quantity for this supply, you need to calculate the number of individual doses required and multiply this by the volume of the dose.

Therefore, you require:

- $3 \times 10 = 30$ doses of 7.5 mL per dose.
- $30 \times 7.5 = 225$ mL.

Therefore, you need to supply a minimum of 225 mL to cover the administration period (not taking into consideration any overage).

**QUESTION 20:** *You are asked to supply a sufficient quantity of inhalers (50 inhalations per inhaler) for the following prescription:*

- *One puff to be inhaled four times a day for 2 months.*

**ANSWER:** To work out the total quantity for this supply, you need to (a) calculate the number of individual doses required and (b) compare this with the number of inhalations in each inhaler.

Therefore, you require:

- $1\times4\times(28\times2)$.
- $4\times56=224$ inhalations.

Therefore, if each inhaler contains 50 inhalations, you will need to supply five inhalers to cover the administration period.

**QUESTION 21:** *You are asked to supply a sufficient quantity of an infusion for the following prescription:*

- *Prepare a 5 mg/1 mL infusion and administer 400 mg over a 3-hour period.*

**ANSWER:** To work out the total quantity of infusion to be prepared, divide the total quantity of drug to be administered by the amount in each volume unit.

In this example, there are 5 mg/1 mL of infusion and we need to administer 400 mg. Therefore, for 400 mg we will need:

- $(400\div5)\times1$ mL of infusion.
- $80\times1=80$ mL of infusion.

Therefore, we need to supply 80 mL of 5 mg/1 mL infusion and administer this over the 3-hour period.

## Questions section 4

If you could not answer or got the wrong answer for any of the questions within section 4, we suggest that as part of your study, you concentrate on the contents of Chapter 5. Specifically:

- Diagnostic Test 1—Question 17—see section 5.1.1.
- Diagnostic Test 1—Question 18—see section 5.2.
- Diagnostic Test 1—Question 19—see section 5.3.
- Diagnostic Test 1—Question 20—see section 5.4.
- Diagnostic Test 1—Question 21—see section 5.5.

FEEDBACK

### Diagnostic calculations test 1

#### Section 5

**QUESTION 22:** *You are asked to make 800 mL pharmaceutical product which contains 2.75% w/v of a drug. How much active ingredient is required?*

**ANSWER:** If the final pharmaceutical product contains 2.75% w/v, this means that there is 2.75 g in every 100 mL of the product. Therefore, in 800 mL of product, there would be:

$$(2.75 \div 100) \times 800 = 22 \, g.$$

Therefore, you will need 22 g of the active ingredient to make 800 mL of a 2.75% w/v pharmaceutical product.

---

**QUESTION 23:** *You are required to make 560 mL of a 1 to 15 solution of a drug (a liquid). How much drug is required?*

**ANSWER:** If the final pharmaceutical product contains 1 to 15 of a drug, this means that there is 1 mL of drug to every 15 mL of solvent (i.e. 1 mL of drug in every 16 mL of product). Therefore, in 560 mL of product, there would be:

$$(560 \div 16) = 35 \, mL.$$

Therefore, you require 35 mL of the drug, diluted with 525 mL $(560 - 35)$ of solvent to make 560 mL of a 1 to 15 solution.

---

**QUESTION 24:** *What is the concentration of a product in percentage which contains a drug in a concentration of 1 in 2.6?*

**ANSWER:** If the concentration of the drug in the preparation is 1 in 2.6, this means that there is 1 part of drug for every 2.6 parts of product. Therefore, to convert to a percentage (either v/v or w/v depending on whether the drug is a liquid or solid, respectively), we need to work out the quantity of the drug (in mL or g) in 100 mL or g of product.

$$(1 \div 2.6) \times 100 = 38.46 \text{ (to two decimal places).}$$

Therefore, a 1 in 2.6 product is the same as a 38.46% product (to two decimal places).

---

**QUESTION 25:** *You are required to make 2.6 L of a 1.25% w/v solution of a drug. How much active ingredient is required?*

**ANSWER:** If the final pharmaceutical product contains 1.25% w/v, this means that there is 1.25 g in every 100 mL of the product. Therefore, in 2600 mL (2.6 L) of product, there would be:

$$(1.25 \div 100) \times 2600 = 32.5 \, g.$$

Therefore, you require 32.5 g of the drug to make 2.6 L of a 1.25% w/v solution.

---

**QUESTION 26:** *You are required to make 225 mL of an 8% w/v solution of a drug from a 10% solution. How much of the more concentrated solution is required?*

**ANSWER:** In this situation, where we are making a particular volume of a solution from a more concentrated solution, we can use the following formula:

$$C_1 V_1 = C_2 V_2$$

In this particular case, the following values apply:

- $C_1 = 10\%$.
- $V_1 = $ Unknown.
- $C_2 = 8\%$.
- $V_2 = 225 \, mL$.

Therefore, entering the values into the equation, you get:

$10 \times V_1 = 8 \times 225.$

$10 \times V_1 = 1800.$

$V_1 = 1800 \div 10.$

$V_1 = 180 \, mL.$

Therefore, you will require 180 mL of a 10% solution of the drug to make 225 mL of an 8% solution.

**QUESTION 27:** *You are asked to produce 200 g of a 5% cream using stock creams of 10% and 2%. How much of each stock cream will you require?*

**ANSWER:** As this question asks for a particular strength of a product to be made, from two other products, one of a higher strength and one of a lower strength, you need to use the alligation grid to calculate the required proportions of each ingredient.

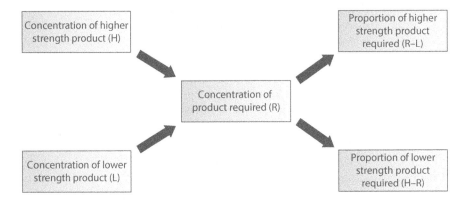

In this particular case, the following values are calculated:

- Proportion of higher strength product required = 5 − 2 = 3.
- Proportion of lower strength product required = 10 − 5 = 5.
- Therefore, the ratio of higher strength to lower strength is 3 to 5.

Then, to calculate the quantity of each ingredient, we need to work out the weight of each part. In total, we require 8 parts (3 + 5) and a total weight of 200 g.

Therefore, each part weighs 200 ÷ 8 = 25 g.

This means that the quantity of the two products to be mixed would be:

Quantity of higher strength product = 3 × 25 = 75 g.

Quantity of lower strength product = 5 × 25 = 125 g.

Therefore, you need to mix 75 g of 10% cream with 125 g of 2% cream to produce 200 g of 5% cream.

## Questions section 5

If you could not answer or got the wrong answer for any of the questions within section 5, we suggest that as part of your study, you concentrate on the contents of Chapter 6. Specifically:

- Diagnostic Test 1—Question 22 —see section 6.2.1.
- Diagnostic Test 1—Question 23 —see section 6.2.2.
- Diagnostic Test 1—Question 24 —see section 6.2.3.
- Diagnostic Test 1—Question 25 —see section 6.3.
- Diagnostic Test 1—Question 26 —see section 6.4.
- Diagnostic Test 1—Question 27 —see section 6.5.

**FEEDBACK**

## Diagnostic calculations test 1

### Section 6

**QUESTION 28:** *You are asked to calculate the amount of a drug required to make 125 mL of infusion where the administration rate is 10 mL/min and the dose is 75 mg/min.*

**ANSWER:** In this case, three pieces of information are available: the required volume of the final solution for infusion, the infusion rate (in volume per set time), and the dose (in quantity of drug per minute). From the latter two pieces of information, it is possible to calculate the strength of the solution.

If the administration rate is 10 mL/min and the dose is 75 mg/min, then the strength of the solution is 75 mg/10 mL.

Once we have calculated the strength of the solution, we can calculate the total quantity of the drug for the required volume.

If there are 75 mg in every 10 mL, in 125 mL there are:

$(75 \div 10) \times 125 = 937.5$ mg.

Therefore, we require 937.5 mg of the drug to make 125 mL of infusion where the administration rate is 10 mL/min and the dose is 75 mg/min.

**QUESTION 29:** *You are asked to calculate the infusion rate, in mL/hour, for a 700 mL solution of a drug at a concentration of 50 mg/25 mL and a required dosage of 350 micrograms/min.*

**ANSWER:** If the dosage is 350 micrograms/min, we need to convert this to volume per hour first as the final administration rate is required in mL/hour.

350 micrograms/min = 350 x 60 = 21 000 micrograms/hour.

21 000 micrograms/hour = 21 mg/hour.

Once we have the administration rate in quantity of drug per hour, we can convert this to the volume of drug to be administered per hour.

The administration rate is 21 mg/hour and the solution has a concentration of 50 mg/25 mL. Therefore, each hour we require:

$(25 \div 50) \times 21 = 10.5$ mL.

Therefore, the infusion rate is 10.5 mL/hour.

**QUESTION 30:** *Calculate the volume of solution required for an infusion of a drug, at a concentration of 75 mg/5 mL, where you are asked to infuse a total of 1500 mg.*

**ANSWER:** If a total of 1500 mg is to be infused, and the concentration of the desired solution is 75 mg/5 mL, the total volume required is:

$$(5 \div 75) \times 1500 = 100 \, \text{mL}.$$

Therefore, we will require a total of 100 mL of a 75 mg/5 mL solution of a drug to infuse a total of 1500 mg.

**QUESTION 31:** *An infusion of a drug is to be delivered at a dose of 5 mg/kg/hour for 6 hours. After this time, the dose is reduced to 3 mg/kg/hour. How long would a 125 mL infusion bag at a concentration of 30 mg/mL last if the patient weighs 70 kg?*

**ANSWER:** To tackle this calculation we first need to work out how much drug will be required for the first 6 hours of infusion. If the dose is 5 mg/kg/hour and the patient weighs 70 kg, the amount of drug infused would be:

$$5 \times 70 \times 6 = 2100 \, \text{mg} \, (2.1 \, \text{g}).$$

Then we need to calculate the volume of infusion that this administration period would require. If there are 30 mg/mL, for 2100 mg, we would infuse:

$$(1 \div 30) \times 2100 = 70 \, \text{mL}.$$

To work out how long the bag will last, we need to calculate the amount of time it will take to use the remainder of the bag after the infusion is reduced to an infusion rate of 3 mg/kg/hour. If the original bag was 125 mL and after 6 hours we have infused 70 mL, the remaining volume will be:

$$125 - 70 = 55 \, \text{mL}.$$

If there are 55 mL remaining and the bag has a concentration of 30 mg/mL, the amount of drug remaining is:

$$(30 \div 1) \times 55 = 1650 \, \text{mg}.$$

At a (revised) administration rate of 3 mg/kg/hour and a patient weight of 70 kg, the revised rate per hour is:

$$3 \times 70 = 210 \, \text{mg/hour}.$$

Therefore, to use the remainder of drug (1650 mg) it will take:

$$1650 \div 210 = 7.86 \, \text{hours (to two decimal places) (7 hours, 51 minutes)}.$$

Therefore, in total, it will take:

$$6 + 7.86 = 13.86 \, \text{hours (to two decimal places) (13 hours, 51 minutes)}.$$

**QUESTION 32:** *A patient requires a dose of 4 mg/hour of a drug. The solution in the syringe is 2 mg/mL and the syringe contains 50 mL and is 10 cm long. At what administration rate, in mm/hour, is the machine required to be set?*

**ANSWER:** Firstly, calculate the volume of drug required per hour. If the dose is 4 mg/hour and the solution is at a concentration of 2 mg/mL, the volume of drug required per hour is:

$$(1 \div 2) \times 4 = 2 \, \text{mL/hour}.$$

Next, work out the length of the syringe that contains this volume. If we consider that the syringe is a fixed cylinder of 50 mL volume and 10 cm length, each cm of length is equivalent to:

$$50 \div 10 = 5 \text{mL/cm}.$$

Therefore, the required 2 mL will be the equivalent of:

$$(1 \div 5) \times 2 = 0.4 \text{cm} \equiv 4 \text{mm}.$$

This means that for a dose of 4 mg/hour of a drug, a 50 mL syringe of 10 cm length containing a solution of 2 mg/mL needs to be set at an administration rate of 4 mm/hour.

**FEEDBACK**

## Questions section 6

If you could not answer or got the wrong answer for any of the questions within section 6, we suggest that as part of your study, you concentrate on the contents of Chapter 7. Specifically:

- Diagnostic Test 1—Question 28—see section 7.2.1.
- Diagnostic Test 1—Question 29—see section 7.2.2.
- Diagnostic Test 1—Question 30—see section 7.2.3.
- Diagnostic Test 1—Question 31—see section 7.3.
- Diagnostic Test 1—Question 32—see section 7.5.1.

### Diagnostic calculations test 1

Section 7

**INSTRUCTIONS**

## The use of calculators for the diagnostic assessment questions in section 7

It is recommended that you undertake the calculations in section 7 using a calculator.

---

**QUESTION 33:**  *Deduce the equation of the straight line given that the gradient of the line is 4.3 and the line passes through the point (8.6,2).*

**ANSWER:**  The equation of the line is: $y = mx + c$ and $m = 4.3$.

Therefore: $y = 4.3x + c$; however, we still need to calculate $c$, and we know when $x = 8.6$, $y = 2$.

$$2 = 4.3 * 8.6 + c, \text{ and thus } c = -34.98.$$

Therefore the equation of the line is $y = 4.3x - 34.98$.

---

**QUESTION 34:**   *Log linearize the following functions:*

   *a)  $y = 10x^2$.*

   *b)  $y = kx^m$.*

   *c)  $y = km^x$.*

   *d)  $C_t = C_0 e^{-kt}$.*

**ANSWER:**   a)  $\log(y) = 1 + 2\log(x)$.

   b)  $\log(y) = \log(k) + m\log(x)$.

   c)  $\log(y) = \log(k) + x\log(m)$.

   d)  $\ln C_t = C_0 - kt$.

**QUESTION 35:**   *To investigate the stability of a drug in solution, the drug concentration is measured over time. The degradation process is shown to follow zero order kinetics. If the initial drug concentration is 100 mg/mL, what concentration will be remaining after 5 days if the rate constant $k_0 = 1.60\,day^{-1}$?*

**ANSWER:**   $C_t = C_0 - k_0 t$.

   $C_t = 100\,mg/mL - 1.60*5$.

   $C_t = 92\,mg/mL$.

**QUESTION 36:**   *In the above example calculate the overage required to ensure a drug concentration of 95 mg/mL after 6 days.*

**ANSWER:**   In this instance we know we want $C_t = 95$ mg/mL after 6 days, so we need to identify what the starting concentration ($C_0$) should be.

   $C_t = C_0 - k_0 t$.

   $95\,mg/mL = C_0 - 1.60*6$.

   $C_0 = 95 + 9.6\,mg/mL = 104.6\,mg/mL$.

   Therefore, an overage of 4.6 mg/mL is required.

**QUESTION 37:**   *Consider the following results from a clinical trial. From the table, calculate the standard error of the mean and the 95% confidence interval for both groups and consider if the results are significantly different.*

| Clinical response Mean (SD) | |
| --- | --- |
| Group A (n=123) | 77.5 (9.6) |
| Group B (n=111) | 61.0 (7.4) |

**ANSWER:**   Group A standard error $= \dfrac{standard\ deviation}{\sqrt{N}}$

   Group A standard error $= \dfrac{9.6}{\sqrt{123}}$

   Standard error $= 0.866$

   Group A 95% CI $= mean \pm (1.96 \times 0.866) = 77.5 \pm (1.70) = 75.5$ to $79.2$

Group B standard error $= \dfrac{7.4}{\sqrt{111}}$

Standard error $= 0.70$

95% CI $= 61.0 \pm (1.96 \times 0.70) = 61.0 \pm 1.37 = 59.6$ to $62.4$

In this study the confidence intervals do not overlap suggesting these results are significantly different.

FEEDBACK

### Questions section 7

If you could not answer or got the wrong answer for any of the questions within section 7, we suggest that as part of your study, you concentrate on the contents of Chapter 8. Specifically:

- Diagnostic Test 1—Question 33—see section 8.3.1.
- Diagnostic Test 1—Question 34—see section 8.3.2.
- Diagnostic Test 1—Question 35—see section 8.4.
- Diagnostic Test 1—Question 36—see section 8.4.1.
- Diagnostic Test 1—Question 37—see section 8.5.

## 1.5 Running case studies: meet the patients

In this section, we meet the patients that you will encounter in the case study questions in the core chapters of the book.

### THE JONES FAMILY

**Mary Jones**

Mary is 35 and is married to John whom she met when she was at school. They have two children, Evie who is 4 years old and George who is 2. Mary works part-time in her local supermarket, a job she doesn't really like but one which works well with her availability in relation to her child-care responsibilities. She weighs 85 kg and is 1.76 m tall. Before having children she was quite active playing both badminton and squash on a regular basis. However, after having her second child, and with her part-time job, her exercise levels have reduced markedly.

**John Jones**

John is Mary's husband and father to Evie and George. John is 37 and is a reasonably heavy smoker. He works full-time as a long-distance lorry driver, weighs 80 kg and is 1.82 m tall. John still keeps reasonably active by playing football every Sunday. When he is not working, spending time with his family or playing football, John likes to go out with his friends to the pub or local curry house.

### Evie Jones

Evie is 4 years old and has recently started at her local school. She weighs 16.5 kg. Evie's best friend is Emma, although she is a sociable child and makes friends easily.

### George Jones

George is Evie's younger brother and is 2 years old. He weighs 13.7 kg. He goes to a local child-minder when his mother is at her part-time job, but he doesn't really like going there.

## OTHER INDIVIDUALS

### Emma

Emma is Evie's school friend. She is also 4 and weighs 20.4 kg. Emma takes medication to treat asthma, which she has had for a couple of years. Emma is an only child and lives with her parents a few doors down from Evie.

### Bob

Bob lives in the same street as the Jones family. Bob has type 2 diabetes, which was first diagnosed when he was 35. He is now 47, is 1.78 m tall and weighs 87 kg. Bob is a travelling salesman and as such can be away from home for several nights every week.

### Marcus

Marcus is unemployed and has a history of mental illness since his late teens. He currently lives in a homeless hostel in the same town as the Jones family. Marcus is 5 foot 4 inches tall, weighs 9 stone and 8 pounds, and is 26 years old.

### Geoff

Geoff is a carpenter and lives with his wife and four teenage children in a large house opposite the Jones family. Geoff and his family love foreign travel and go abroad whenever they can. Geoff is 48 years old, 12 stone and 6 pounds, and is 6 foot, 1 inch tall.

### Roger

Roger is 85 and lives on his own. He was married but his wife died a couple of years ago. Roger has two daughters who are both married. One lives in Australia, but his other daughter lives only 20 miles away and visits Roger at least once a week for at least an hour. Roger was originally in the army but after he retired from the service he worked at a local supermarket, firstly on the check-out and then latterly as a car park attendant collecting trolleys. Although he enjoyed his job, Roger had to give it up a year ago as it was too much for him. Roger weighs 60.4 kg and is 1.6 m tall.

## 1.6 Diagnostic calculations test 2

This test has been designed to be undertaken after your studies and/or revision on pharmaceutical calculations. It is recommended that you undertake the whole test in one sitting and only use a calculator for those questions where it is stated that it is permitted. Once you have answered all questions, and checked your answers yourself, you can refer to the answers to the questions at the end of this section (see section 1.6.2). Now you have completed your study and/or revision on pharmaceutical calculations, it is hoped that you were able to answer all the questions within this diagnostic calculations test correctly. However, should you have found any of the questions difficult, section 1.6.2 also provides guidance on which chapters and/or sections to refer back to for help answering each question.

### 1.6.1 Diagnostic calculations test

**INSTRUCTIONS**

### The use of calculators during diagnostic calculations test 2

It is recommended that you undertake some of the following calculations within this diagnostic calculations test without the use of a calculator.

Unless stated otherwise, all of the self-assessment questions within this test can be undertaken using a pen and paper.

### Diagnostic calculations test 2

**Section 1**

**QUESTION 1:** What is 0.212 g in milligrams, micrograms, and nanograms?

**QUESTION 2:** What is 486 nanolitres in litres?

**QUESTION 3:** You are asked to make 150 mL pharmaceutical product which contains 9.5% w/v of an active ingredient. How much active ingredient is required?

**QUESTION 4:** You are required to make 650 g of a dusting powder according to the following formula:

- Ingredient A    7 parts.
- Ingredient B    8 parts.
- Ingredient C    1 part.
- Ingredient D    to 25 parts.

What is the weight of each of the powders in the final preparation?

**QUESTION 5:** How much of a liquid ingredient is required for 600 mL of a 1 to 10 solution?

**QUESTION 6:** A patient weighs 10 st and 4 lb. What is the patient's weight in kilograms? (Note: there are approximately 2.2 pounds in a kilogram.)

## Diagnostic calculations test 2

### Section 2

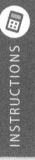

### The use of calculators for the diagnostic assessment questions in section 2

It is recommended that you undertake the calculations in section 2 using a calculator.

INSTRUCTIONS

**QUESTION 7:**   *How many significant figures do the following values contain?*

    *a)* *1908.32.*

    *b)* *0.009.*

    *c)* *0.5005.*

    *d)* *120.1.*

**QUESTION 8:**   *The total weight of vancomycin and its container is $78 \pm 0.2$ g. After removal of the drug, the container had a weight of $0.18 \pm 0.1$ g. What is the weight of vancomycin that was in the container?*

**QUESTION 9:**   *In an experiment you weigh out 5.27 g of drug on a two decimal place balance and dissolve this completely in $100 \pm 0.5$ mL of water. Using the propagation of uncertainty technique, what is the uncertainty associated with the weight of the drug and the resultant drug solution?*

**QUESTION 10:**   *A 100 mL antibiotic suspension was prepared to contain 250 mg of drug. Analysis of the contents determined that the suspension contained 244 mg of drug. What was the absolute error, the relative error, and percentage relative error associated with this measurement?*

**QUESTION 11:**   *The drug concentration of five capsules was measured:*

    *Drug concentration (in mg): 113, 111, 117, 114, 117.*

    *Calculate the following (assume this is a sample data set):*

    *a)* *Mean, median, mode.*

    *b)* *Mean deviation.*

    *c)* *Variance.*

    *d)* *Standard deviation.*

    *e)* *Standard error.*

    *f)* *% coefficient of variation.*

## Diagnostic calculations test 2

### Section 3

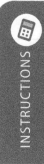

INSTRUCTIONS

### The use of calculators for the diagnostic assessment questions in section 3

It is recommended that you undertake the calculations in section 3 using a calculator.

**QUESTION 12:** *Cefuroxime, when reconstituted with 1.84 mL of water for injection, gives a solution of 200 mg in 2 mL. What is the displacement volume for cefuroxime?*

**QUESTION 13:** *Aspirin has a displacement value in theobroma oil of 1.1. If a suppository is to contain 0.3 g of aspirin, calculate what weight of drug and glycol gelatin will be needed to prepare six suppositories using a nominal 2 g mould. Assume that a nominal 1 g mould will hold 1.2 g of glycol gelatin base.*

**QUESTION 14:** *Calculate how much NaCl is required to make a 20 mL bottle of 1% chloramphenicol eye drops isotonic, given that 1% w/v of chloramphenicol solution freezes at –0.06°C and a 1% w/v of NaCl solution freezes at –0.576°C. An isotonic solution freezes at –0.52°C.*

**QUESTION 15:** *What mass of KCl is required to produce 200 mL of a solution that is isotonic with blood. The MW of KCl = 74.5. The osmolarity of blood = 0.3 mol/L.*

**QUESTION 16:** *How much sodium chloride is required to make 100 mL of a 2% w/v solution of pilocarpine nitrate isotonic? (Sodium chloride equivalent of pilocarpine nitrate is 0.22.)*

## Diagnostic calculations test 2

### Section 4

**QUESTION 17:** *You are asked to arrange a two-month supply of medication where the patient has been advised to take two capsules in the morning, one at lunchtime and one in the evening. How many capsules are required?*

**QUESTION 18:** *You are asked to supply the following course of prednisolone 5 mg tablets to cover a period of 28 days:*

- *6 OD 1/7.*
- *5 OD 1/7.*
- *4 OD 2/7.*
- *3 OD 2/7.*
- *2 OD 2/7.*
- *1 OD thereafter.*

*How many tablets should you supply?*

**QUESTION 19:**   *You are asked to supply a sufficient quantity of ointment (120 g of ointment per container) for the following prescription:*

   • *Apply to the scalp twice a day for 2 weeks.*

*The* British National Formulary[1] *advises that for creams and ointments applied to the scalp, 50-100 g would be required for a week of twice-daily applications.*

**QUESTION 20:**   *You are asked to supply a sufficient quantity of an infusion for the following prescription:*

   • *Prepare an 8 mg/10 mL infusion and administer 400 mg over a 30-minute period.*

**QUESTION 21:**   *You are asked to supply an antibiotic mixture for a 2-year-old patient according to the following prescription:*

   • *5 mL to be given twice a day for 10 days.*

*Once reconstituted, each container will contain 140 mL of liquid and will last for 14 days.*

## Diagnostic calculations test 2

### Section 5

**QUESTION 22:**   *You are asked to make 235 mL pharmaceutical product which contains 1.9% v/v of a drug. How much active ingredient is required?*

**QUESTION 23:**   *You are required to make 250 mL of a 1 in 50 solution of a drug (a solid). How much drug is required?*

**QUESTION 24:**   *A drug, a liquid, is dissolved in water producing a 1 to 9 solution. What is the equivalent strength expressed as % v/v?*

**QUESTION 25:**   *You are required to make 240 mL of a 14% w/v solution of a drug (a solid). How much active ingredient is required?*

**QUESTION 26:**   *You are told that 268 mL of a 19% w/v solution of a drug was used to make 900 mL of final solution. What is the concentration of this final solution?*

**QUESTION 27:**   *You are asked to produce 250 g of a 9.5% cream using stock cream of 2% and the active ingredient. How much of the stock cream and the active ingredient will you require?*

## Diagnostic calculations test 2

### Section 6

**QUESTION 28:**   *You are asked to calculate the amount of a solution of a drug required to make 300 mL of infusion where the administration rate is 1.5 mL/min and the dose is 750 micrograms/min. The solution of drug is 25 mg/5 mL.*

**QUESTION 29:**   *You are asked to calculate the amount of a drug required to make 1 L of infusion where the administration rate is 10 mL/min and the dose is 15 micrograms/kg/min. The patient weighs 80 kg.*

**QUESTION 30:**   *An infusion of a drug is to be delivered at a dose of 3 mg/kg/hour for 4 hours. After this time, the dose is increased to 5 mg/kg/hour. After the change of administration rate, how long would it take for the remainder of a 500 mL infusion bag at a concentration of 15 mg/mL to be administered if the patient weighs 75 kg?*

**QUESTION 31:** *A patient currently takes 30 mg of oral morphine twice a day (as sustained release tablets). His doctor wants to change this to an intramuscular administration of diamorphine. What is the total daily dose of intramuscular (IM) diamorphine required? (Note: you will need to use the* British National Formulary *to answer this question.)*

**QUESTION 32:** *A patient requires a dose of 800 mg/hour of a drug. The solution in the infusion bag is 10 mg/mL and the bag contains 750 mL. The bag is set up on a giving set with a drop volume of 0.1 mL. At what drop rate (drops per minute) does the giving set need to be set?*

## Diagnostic calculations test 2

### Section 7

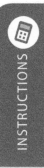

**INSTRUCTIONS**

## The use of calculators for the diagnostic assessment questions in section 7

It is recommended that you undertake the calculations in section 7 using a calculator.

**QUESTION 33:** *The following equations each represent a straight-line plot on a graph. From the equations, identify the gradient and the y intercept for each.*

    *a)* $y = 27x - 5.3$.

    *b)* $y = 0.12x$.

    *c)* $\ln[H^+] = -2.303pH$ *(where* $\ln[H^+]$ *is plotted against pH).*

    *d)* $\ln(y) = 2.06 - 0.31x$.

**QUESTION 34:** *Log linearize the following functions:*

    *a)* $y = 100x^{-7}$.

    *b)* $y = e^{-2x}$.

    *c)* $y = 3^x$.

    *d)* $C_t = 6e^{-5t}$.

**QUESTION 35:** *A drug is shown to degrade by first order rate kinetics. If the rate constant* $k_1 = 0.004\ day^{-1}$*, what percentage of drug will remain after 15 days?*

**QUESTION 36:** *In the above example, calculate the overage required to ensure a drug concentration of 95 mg/mL after 30 days.*

**QUESTION 37:** *Consider the following results in the comparison of a new drug and placebo in the reduction of blood pressure in a study. Use the 95% confidence intervals to determine if the differences seen are significant.*

| | % Number of cases of reduced blood pressure (95% CI) |
|---|---|
| Group receiving new drug | 8.8% (8.0−9.1) |
| Placebo group | 7.1% (6.2−7.7) |

## 1.6.2 Answers to diagnostic calculations test

This section contains the worked answers for diagnostic calculations test 2.

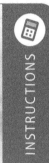

### The use of calculators during diagnostic calculations test 2

It is recommended that you undertake some of the following calculations within this diagnostic calculations test without the use of a calculator.

Unless stated otherwise, all of the self-assessment questions within this test can be undertaken using a pen and paper.

INSTRUCTIONS

### Diagnostic calculations test 2

#### Section 1

**QUESTION 1:** *What is 0.212 g in milligrams, micrograms, and nanograms?*

**ANSWER:** This calculation involves moving down the weight units in multiples of 1000. Therefore:

0.212 g in milligrams = 0.212 × 1000 = 212 mg.

Continuing down the weight units, we can move from milligrams to micrograms by multiplying by another 1000.

212 mg (0.212 g) in micrograms = 212 × 1000 = 212 000 micrograms.

Continuing down the weight units, we can move from micrograms to nanograms by multiplying by another 1000.

212 000 micrograms (212 mg; 0.212 g) in nanograms
= 212 000 × 1000 = 212 000 000 nanograms.

**QUESTION 2:** *What is 486 nanolitres in litres?*

**ANSWER:** This calculation involves moving up the volume units in multiples of 1000. However, in this case, the question asks for the answer in litres, without reporting the intermediate units (i.e. the microlitres and the millilitres). Rather than moving straight from nanolitres to litres, it is suggested that you attempt the question in stages, moving through the intermediary units. Therefore:

486 nanolitres in microlitres = 486 ÷ 1000 = 0.486 microlitres.

Continuing up the volume units, we can move from microlitres to millilitres by dividing by another 1000.

0.486 microlitres (486 nanolitres) in millilitres

$=0.486 \div 1000 = 0.000486\,mL.$

Continuing up the volume units, we can move from millilitres to litres by dividing by another 1000.

0.000486 mL (486 nanolitres; 0.486 microlitres)

$=0.000486 \div 1000 = 0.000000486\,L.$

---

**QUESTION 3:** *You are asked to make 150 mL pharmaceutical product which contains 9.5% w/v of an active ingredient. How much active ingredient is required?*

**ANSWER:** If the final pharmaceutical product contains 9.5% w/v, this means that there are 9.5 g in every 100 mL of the product. Therefore, in 150 mL of product, there would be:

$(9.5 \div 100) \times 150 = 14.25\,g.$

Therefore, you will need 14.25 g of active ingredient to make 150 mL of a 9.5% w/v pharmaceutical product.

---

**QUESTION 4:** *You are required to make 650 g of a dusting powder according to the following formula:*

- *Ingredient A    7 parts.*
- *Ingredient B    8 parts.*
- *Ingredient C    1 part.*
- *Ingredient D    to 25 parts.*

*What is the weight of each of the powders in the final preparation?*

**ANSWER:** The formula indicates that for every 25 parts of preparation, Ingredient A accounts for 7 parts, Ingredient B accounts for 8 parts, and Ingredient C accounts for 1 part. Therefore, Ingredient D accounts for:

$25 - (7 + 8 + 1) = 9$ parts.

Therefore, the formula for the amount of each ingredient would be the total weight of the dusting powder (650 g) divided by the total number of parts (25), then multiplied by the number of parts of that ingredient (Ingredient A, 7 parts; Ingredient B, 8 parts; Ingredient C, 1 part; Ingredient D, 9 parts).

This means that in 650 g of the dusting powder, there are the following amounts of each ingredient:

- Ingredient A    $(650 \div 25) \times 7 = 182\,g.$
- Ingredient B    $(650 \div 25) \times 8 = 208\,g.$
- Ingredient C    $(650 \div 25) \times 1 = 26\,g.$
- Ingredient D    $(650 \div 25) \times 9 = 234\,g.$

To check this calculation, add up the amounts of the individual ingredients and check that they total 650 g.

$182 + 208 + 26 + 234 = 650\,g.$

**QUESTION 5:** *How much of a liquid ingredient is required for 600 mL of a 1 to 10 solution?*

**ANSWER:** If the solute is to be added to form a 1 to 10 solution, this means that for every 11 mL of solution (10 + 1), 1 mL will be solute. Therefore in 600 mL, there will be:

$600 \div 11 = 54.55$ mL of the liquid ingredient (to two decimal places).

Therefore, we require 54.55 mL of the ingredient and dissolve this in $(600 - 54.55) = 545.45$ mL of solvent.

---

**QUESTION 6:** *A patient weighs 10 st and 4 lb. What is the patient's weight in kilograms? (Note: there are approximately 2.2 pounds in a kilogram.)*

**ANSWER** If 2.2 lb = 1 kg, we need to know the patient's weight in pounds. We can convert the patient's weight of 10 st 4 lb into pounds as follows:

$(10 \times 14) + 4 = 144$ lb.

If 2.2 lb = 1 kg, 144 lb is the same as:

$144 \div 2.2 = 65.45$ kg (to two decimal places).

---

## Questions section 1

If you could not answer or got the wrong answer for any of the questions within section 1, we suggest that you revisit the contents of Chapter 2. Specifically:

- Diagnostic Test 2—Question 1—see section 2.2.1.
- Diagnostic Test 2—Question 2—see section 2.2.2.
- Diagnostic Test 2—Question 3—see section 2.3.1.
- Diagnostic Test 2—Question 4—see section 2.3.3.
- Diagnostic Test 2—Question 5—see section 2.3.4.
- Diagnostic Test 2—Question 6—see section 2.5.2.

FEEDBACK

### Diagnostic calculations test 2

Section 2

## The use of calculators for the diagnostic assessment questions in section 2

It is recommended that you undertake the calculations in section 2 using a calculator.

INSTRUCTIONS

**QUESTION 7:** *How many significant figures do the following values contain?*

  *a) 1908.32.*

  *b) 0.009.*

  *c) 0.5005.*

  *d) 120.1.*

**ANSWER:** Count from the first non-zero value:

  a) 1908.32 (6 significant figures).

  b) 0.009 (1 significant figure).

  c) 0.5005 (4 significant figures).

  d) 120.1 (4 significant figures).

**QUESTION 8:** *The total weight of vancomycin and its container is 78±0.2 g. After removal of the drug, the container had a weight of 0.18±0.1 g. What is the weight of vancomycin that was in the container?*

**ANSWER:** 77.8±0.2 g.

**QUESTION 9:** *In an experiment you weigh out 5.27 g of drug on a two decimal place balance and dissolve this completely in 100±0.5 mL of water. Using the propagation of uncertainty technique, what is the uncertainty associated with the weight of the drug and the resultant drug solution?*

**ANSWER:** The uncertainty of the drug mass is 0.005 g and therefore the resulting solution has a concentration of 52.7±0.27 mg/mL.

**QUESTION 10:** *A 100 mL antibiotic suspension was prepared to contain 250 mg of drug. Analysis of the contents determined that the suspension contained 244 mg of drug. What was the absolute error, the relative error, and percentage relative error associated with this measurement?*

**ANSWER:** The absolute error is 6 mg, the relative error is 0.024 and the percentage relative error is 2.4%.

**QUESTION 11:** *The drug concentration of five capsules was measured:*

  *Drug concentration (in mg): 113, 111, 117, 114, 117.*

  *Calculate the following (assume this is a sample data set):*

  *a) Mean, median, mode.*

  *b) Mean deviation.*

  *c) Variance.*

  *d) Standard deviation.*

  *e) Standard error.*

  *f) % coefficient of variation.*

**ANSWER:**

  a) Mean=114.4 mg, median=114 mg, mode=117 mg.

  b) Mean deviation=2.08 mg.

  c) Variance=6.80.

  d) Standard deviation=2.61 mg.

  e) Standard error=1.17 mg.

  f) % coefficient of variation=2.28%.

## Questions section 2

If you could not answer or got the wrong answer for any of the questions within section 2, we suggest that you revisit the contents of Chapter 3. Specifically:

- Diagnostic Test 2—Question 7—see section 3.2.1.
- Diagnostic Test 2—Question 8—see section 3.2.2.
- Diagnostic Test 2—Question 9—see section 3.2.2.
- Diagnostic Test 2—Question 10—see section 3.3.1.
- Diagnostic Test 2—Question 11—see section 3.5.

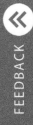

FEEDBACK

## Diagnostic calculations test 2

### Section 3

## The use of calculators for the diagnostic assessment questions in section 3

It is recommended that you undertake the calculations in section 3 using a calculator.

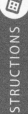

INSTRUCTIONS

---

**QUESTION 12:** *Cefuroxime, when reconstituted with 1.84 mL of water for injection, gives a solution of 200 mg in 2 mL. What is the displacement volume for cefuroxime?*

**ANSWER:** The displacement volume is 0.16 mL/200 mg.

---

**QUESTION 13:** *Aspirin has a displacement value in theobroma oil of 1.1. If a suppository is to contain 0.3 g of aspirin, calculate what weight of drug and glycol gelatin will be needed to prepare six suppositories using a nominal 2 g mould. Assume that a nominal 1 g mould will hold 1.2 g of glycol gelatin base.*

**ANSWER:** Amount of drug required = 1.8 g.

Total amount of theobroma base = 10.36 g.

Total amount of glycol gelatin base = 12.43 g.

---

**QUESTION 14:** *Calculate how much NaCl is required to make a 20 mL bottle of 1% chloramphenicol eye drops isotonic given that 1% w/v of chloramphenicol solution freezes at −0.06°C and a 1% w/v of NaCl solution freezes at −0.576°C. An isotonic solution freezes at −0.52°C.*

**ANSWER:** 0.80% w/v of NaCl is required; therefore for 20 mL, 0.16 g of NaCl is required.

---

**QUESTION 15:**  *What mass of KCl is required to produce 200 mL of a solution that is isotonic with blood. The MW of KCl = 74.5. The osmolarity of blood = 0.3 mol/L.*

**ANSWER:**  200 mL will require 2.24 g of KCl.

**QUESTION 16:**  *How much sodium chloride is required to make 100 mL of a 2% w/v solution of pilocarpine nitrate isotonic? (Sodium chloride equivalent of pilocarpine nitrate is 0.22.)*

**ANSWER:**  0.46 g of sodium chloride per 100 mL of 2% solution of pilocarpine nitrate is required to make the solution isotonic.

FEEDBACK

### Questions section 3

If you could not answer or got the wrong answer for any of the questions within section 3, we suggest that you revisit the contents of Chapter 4. Specifically:

- Diagnostic Test 2—Question 12—see section 4.2.1.
- Diagnostic Test 2—Question 13—see section 4.2.2.
- Diagnostic Test 2—Question 14—see section 4.4.1.
- Diagnostic Test 2—Question 15—see section 4.4.2.
- Diagnostic Test 2—Question 16—see section 4.4.4.

### Diagnostic calculations test 2

#### Section 4

**QUESTION 17:**  *You are asked to arrange a two-month supply of medication where the patient has been advised to take two capsules in the morning, one at lunchtime and one in the evening. How many capsules are required?*

**ANSWER:**  In this case, there is no additional information as to the amount of medication to be supplied and so each month can be taken to be 28 days.

For a two-month supply:

- Each day, the patient will take $2+1+1=4$ capsules.
- Therefore, in a pharmaceutical month the patient will take $4 \times 28 = 112$ capsules.
- Therefore, in 2 months, the patient will take $112 \times 2 = 224$.

Therefore, you need to supply 224 capsules to cover the two-month course of medication.

**QUESTION 18:**  *You are asked to supply the following course of prednisolone 5 mg tablets to cover a period of 28 days:*

- *6 OD 1/7.*
- *5 OD 1/7.*
- *4 OD 2/7.*
- *3 OD 2/7.*

- *2 OD 2/7.*
- *1 OD thereafter.*

*How many tablets should you supply?*

ANSWER:    This is a reducing dose of 5 mg prednisolone tablets. The best way to work out the total number of tablets to be supplied is to work it out on a day-by-day basis:

This works out as follows:

- 6 daily for 1 day = 6 tablets.
- 5 daily for 1 day = 5 tablets.
- 4 daily for 2 days = 8 tablets.
- 3 daily for 2 days = 6 tablets.
- 2 daily for 2 days = 4 tablets.
- 1 daily for the remaining number of days = $1 \times (28 - 8) = 20$ tablets.

Therefore, the total is 49 tablets.

Therefore, you need to supply 49 tablets to cover the entire reducing course of the 5 mg prednisolone tablets.

---

QUESTION 19:    *You are asked to supply a sufficient quantity of ointment (120 g of ointment per container) for the following prescription:*

- *Apply to the scalp twice a day for 2 weeks.*

*The* British National Formulary[2] *advises that for creams and ointments applied to the scalp, 50-100 g would be required for a week of twice-daily applications.*

ANSWER:    To work out the total quantity for this supply, you need to (a) calculate the amount of cream required for each administration and (b) multiply this by the administration period.

According to the *British National Formulary*, the amount of cream required for twice-daily administration to the scalp for a week is:

- 50-100 g.

Then, you need to multiply this by two for the required administration period (2 weeks), giving the required amount as:

- 100-200 g.

Therefore, if the cream is packaged in 120 g containers, you need to supply one or two containers depending on the patient's usage within the application range.

---

QUESTION 20:    *You are asked to supply a sufficient quantity of an infusion for the following prescription:*

- *Prepare an 8 mg/10 mL infusion and administer 400 mg over a 30-minute period.*

ANSWER:    To work out the total quantity of infusion to be prepared, divide the total quantity of drug to be administered by the amount in each volume unit.

---

2 *British National Formulary* 67th Edition, Section 13.1.2, page 764.

In this example, there are 8 mg/10 mL of infusion and we need to administer 400 mg. Therefore, for 400 mg we will need:

- $(400 \div 8) \times 10$ mL of infusion.
- $50 \times 10 = 500$ mL of infusion.

Therefore, we need to supply 500 mL of 8 mg/10 mL infusion and administer this over the 30-minute period.

**QUESTION 21:** *You are asked to supply a sufficient quantity of an antibiotic mixture for a 2-year-old patient according to the following prescription:*

- *5 mL to be given twice a day for 10 days.*

*Once reconstituted, each container will contain 140 mL of liquid and will last for 14 days.*

**ANSWER:** To work out the total quantity for this supply, you need to calculate the number of individual doses required and multiply this by the volume of the dose.

Therefore, you require:

- $10 \times 2 = 20$ doses of 5 mL per dose.
- $20 \times 5 = 100$ mL.

Therefore, you need to supply a minimum of 100 mL to cover the administration period (not taking into consideration any overage).

However, it is noted that the reconstituted medication comes in multiples of 140 mL and will expire 14 days following reconstitution.

Therefore, you will be able to supply $1 \times 140$ mL (to cover the required 100 mL). Although the reconstituted product will expire in 14 days, this is longer than the length of the course (10 days), and so does not cause a problem. In addition, the supply of 140 mL will take account of any overage required (as the total supply will be for 140 mL, with a requirement of 100 mL for the 10-day course).

FEEDBACK

## Questions section 4

If you could not answer or got the wrong answer for any of the questions within section 4, we suggest that you revisit the contents of Chapter 5. Specifically:

- Diagnostic Test 2—Question 17—see section 5.1.1.
- Diagnostic Test 2—Question 18—see section 5.2.
- Diagnostic Test 2—Question 19—see section 5.4.
- Diagnostic Test 2—Question 20—see section 5.5.
- Diagnostic Test 2—Question 21—see section 5.6.

## Diagnostic calculations test 2

### Section 5

**QUESTION 22:** *You are asked to make 235 mL pharmaceutical product which contains 1.9% v/v of a drug. How much active ingredient is required?*

**ANSWER:** If the final pharmaceutical product contains 1.9% w/v, this means that there is 1.9 g in every 100 mL of the product. Therefore, in 235 mL of product, there would be:

$$(1.9 \div 100) \times 235 = 4.465\,g.$$

Therefore, you will need 4.465 g of the drug to make 235 mL of a 1.9% w/v pharmaceutical product.

**QUESTION 23:** *You are required to make 250 mL of a 1 in 50 solution of a drug (a solid). How much drug is required?*

**ANSWER:** If the final pharmaceutical product contains 1 in 50 of a drug, this means that there is 1 g of the drug in every 50 mL of product. Therefore, in 250 mL of product, there would be:

$$(250 \div 50) = 5\,g.$$

Therefore, you require 5 g of the drug make 250 mL of a 1 in 50 solution.

**QUESTION 24:** *A drug, a liquid, is dissolved in water producing a 1 to 9 solution. What is the equivalent strength expressed as % v/v?*

**ANSWER:** If the concentration of the drug in the preparation is 1 to 9, this means that there is 1 mL of drug to every 9 mL of water (i.e. a total of 10 mL). Therefore, to convert to a percentage (v/v), we need to work out the quantity of the drug (in mL) in 100 mL of product.

$$(1 \div 10) \times 100 = 10.$$

Therefore, a 1 to 9 product is the same as a 10% v/v product.

**QUESTION 25:** *You are required to make 240 mL of a 14% w/v solution of a drug (a solid). How much active ingredient is required?*

**ANSWER:** If the final pharmaceutical product contains 14% w/v, this means that there are 14 g in every 100 mL of the product. Therefore, in 240 mL of product, there would be:

$$(14 \div 100) \times 240 = 33.6\,g.$$

Therefore, you require 33.6 g of the drug to make 240 mL of a 14% w/v solution.

**QUESTION 26:** *You are told that 268 mL of a 19% w/v solution of a drug was used to make 900 mL of a final solution. What is the concentration of this final solution?*

**ANSWER:** Where we are making a particular volume of a solution from a more concentrated solution, we can use the following formula:

$$C_1 V_1 = C_2 V_2$$

In this particular case, the following values apply:

- $C_1 = 19\%$.
- $V_1 = 268\,mL$.

- $C_2$ = Unknown.
- $V_2$ = 900 mL.

Therefore, entering the values into the equation, you get:

$19 \times 268 = C_2 \times 900$.

$5092 = C_2 \times 900$.

$C_2 = 5092 \div 900$.

$C_2 = 5.66\%$ (to two decimal places).

Therefore, you will produce a 5.66% solution (to two decimal places) by diluting 268 mL of a 19% solution of a drug to 900 mL.

**QUESTION 27:** *You are asked to produce 250 g of a 9.5% cream using stock cream of 2% and the active ingredient. How much of the stock cream and the active ingredient will you require?*

**ANSWER:** As this question asks for a particular strength of a product to be made, from two other products, the active ingredient and a product of a lower strength, you need to use the alligation grid to calculate the required proportions of each ingredient.

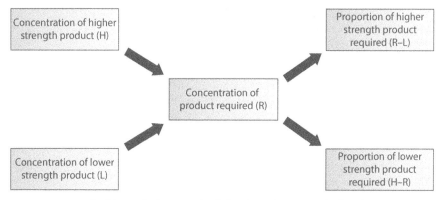

In this particular case, the following values are calculated:

- Proportion of higher strength product required = 9.5 − 2 = 7.5.
- Proportion of lower strength product required = 100 − 9.5 = 90.5.
- Therefore, the ratio of higher strength to lower strength is 7.5 to 90.5.

Then, to calculate the quantity of each ingredient, we need to work out the weight of each part. In total, we require 98 parts (7.5 + 90.5) and a total weight of 250 g.

Therefore, each part weighs 250 ÷ 98 = 2.55 g (to two decimal places).

This means that the quantity of the two products to be mixed would be:

Quantity of active ingredient = 7.5 × (250 ÷ 98) = 19.13 g (to two decimal places).

Quantity of lower strength product = 90.5 × (250 ÷ 98) = 230.87 g (to two decimal places).

Therefore, you need to mix 230.87 g of 2% cream with 19.13 g of active ingredient to produce 250 g of 9.5% cream.

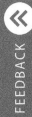

## Questions section 5

If you could not answer or got the wrong answer for any of the questions within section 5, we suggest that you revisit the contents of Chapter 6. Specifically:

- Diagnostic Test 2—Question 22—see section 6.2.1.
- Diagnostic Test 2—Question 23—see section 6.2.2.
- Diagnostic Test 2—Question 24—see section 6.2.3.
- Diagnostic Test 2—Question 25—see section 6.3.
- Diagnostic Test 2—Question 26—see section 6.4.
- Diagnostic Test 2—Question 27—see section 6.5.

FEEDBACK

## Diagnostic calculations test 2

### Section 6

**QUESTION 28:** *You are asked to calculate the amount of a solution of a drug required to make 300 mL of infusion where the administration rate is 1.5 mL/min and the dose is 750 micrograms/min. The solution of drug is 25 mg/5 mL.*

**ANSWER:** Three pieces of information are available: the required volume of the final solution for infusion, the infusion rate (in volume per set time), and the dose (in quantity of drug per minute). In addition, the strength of the concentrated solution to be used is also provided. From the infusion rate and dose, it is possible to calculate the strength of the solution.

If the administration rate is 1.5 mL/min and the dose is 750 micrograms/min, then the strength of the solution is 750 micrograms/1.5 mL.

Once we have calculated the strength of the solution, we can calculate the total quantity of drug for the required volume.

If there are 750 micrograms in every 1.5 mL, in 300 mL there are:

$$(750 \div 1.5) \times 300 = 150\,000 \text{ micrograms} \equiv 150 \text{ mg.}$$

Therefore, we require 150 mg of drug to make 300 mL of infusion where the administration rate is 1.5 mL/min and the dose is 750 micrograms/min.

In this case the drug is coming from a more concentrated solution. Therefore, we need to calculate the volume of this solution required to provide the correct quantity of drug.

If the solution contains 25 mg/5 mL, for 150 mg, we require:

$$(5 \div 25) \times 150 = 30 \text{ mL.}$$

Therefore, we need to add 30 mL of the 25 mg/5 mL to a 300 mL infusion bag (remembering to remove a corresponding 30 mL first to maintain the final volume at 300 mL) to make 300 mL of infusion where the administration rate is 1.5 mL/min and the dose is 750 micrograms/min.

**QUESTION 29:** *You are asked to calculate the amount of a drug required to make 1 L of infusion where the administration rate is 10 mL/min and the dose is 15 micrograms/kg/min. The patient weighs 80 kg.*

**ANSWER:**     Three pieces of information are available: the required volume of the final solution for infusion, the infusion rate (in volume per set time), and the dose (in quantity of drug per kilogram of patient per minute). From the latter two pieces of information, it is possible to calculate the strength of the solution once the dosage has been converted from weight of drug per kilogram of patient per minute to the total weight of drug to be administered per minute.

Firstly, convert the dosage using the patient's weight:

If the dosage is 15 micrograms/kg/min and the patient weighs 80 kg, the dose is:

$15 \times 80 = 1200$ micrograms/min $\equiv 1.2$ mg/min.

If the administration rate is 10 mL/min and the dose is 1.2 mg/min, then the strength of the solution is 1.2 mg/10 mL.

Once we have calculated the strength of the solution, we can calculate the total quantity of drug for the required volume.

If there are 1.2 mg in every 10 mL, in 1 L (1000 mL) there are:

$(1.2 \div 10) \times 1000 = 120$ mg.

Therefore, we require 120 mg of drug to make 1 L of infusion where the administration rate is 10 mL/min and the dose is 15 micrograms/kg/min for an 80 kg patient.

**QUESTION 30:**    *An infusion of a drug is to be delivered at a dose of 3 mg/kg/hour for 4 hours. After this time, the dose is increased to 5 mg/kg/hour. After the change of administration rate, how long would it take for the remainder of a 500 mL infusion bag at a concentration of 15 mg/mL to be administered if the patient weighs 75 kg?*

**ANSWER:**    To tackle this calculation we first need to work out how much drug will be required for the first 4 hours of infusion. If the dose is 3 mg/kg/hour and the patient weighs 75 kg, the amount of drug infused would be:

$3 \times 75 \times 4 = 900$ mg.

Then we need to calculate the volume of infusion that this administration period would require. If there are 15 mg/mL, for 900 mg, we would infuse:

$(1 \div 15) \times 900 = 60$ mL.

To work out how long the remainder of the bag will last, we need to calculate the amount of time it will take to use the remainder of the bag after the infusion is increased to an infusion rate of 5 mg/kg/hour. If the original bag was 500 mL and after 4 hours we have infused 60 mL, the remaining volume will be:

$500 - 60 = 440$ mL.

If there are 440 mL remaining and the bag has a concentration of 15 mg/mL, the amount of drug remaining is:

$(15 \div 1) \times 440 = 6600$ mg (6.6 g).

At a (revised) administration rate of 5 mg/kg/hour and a patient weight of 75 kg, the revised rate per hour is:

$5 \times 75 = 375$ mg/hour.

Therefore, to use the remainder of drug (6600 mg) it will take:

$6600 \div 375 = 17.6$ hours $\equiv$ 17 hours, 36 minutes.

Therefore, after the end of the first administration period it will take a further 17 hours and 36 minutes to administer the remainder of the infusion.

---

**QUESTION 31:** *A patient currently takes 30 mg of oral morphine twice a day (as sustained release tablets). His doctor wants to change this to an intramuscular administration of diamorphine. What is the total daily dose of intramuscular (IM) diamorphine required? (Note: you will need to use the* British National Formulary *to answer this question.)*

**ANSWER:** To convert oral morphine to intramuscular diamorphine, you need to consult the equivalent dosage table in the *British National Formulary* (see *Prescribing in palliative care*). This states that the equivalent dose of IM diamorphine is approximately one-third of the oral dose of morphine. Therefore, a twice-daily dose of 30 mg oral morphine is equivalent to:

$(30 \times 2) \div 3 = 20$ mg.

Therefore, the total daily dose of IM diamorphine required is 20 mg.

---

**QUESTION 32:** *A patient requires a dose of 800 mg/hour of a drug. The solution in the infusion bag is 10 mg/mL and the bag contains 750 mL. The bag is set up on a giving set with a drop volume of 0.1 mL. At what drop rate (drops per minute) does the giving set need to be set?*

**ANSWER:** Firstly, calculate the volume of drug required per minute. If the dose is 800 mg/hour and the solution is at a concentration of 10 mg/mL, the volume of drug required per hour is:

$(1 \div 10) \times 800 = 80$ mL/hour.

Next, convert this to a volume per minute.

$80 \div 60 = 1.33$ mL/min (to two decimal places).

Then convert this volume to drops, based on each drop having a volume of 0.1 mL.

$(80 \div 60) \div 0.1 = 13.33$ drops per minute (to two decimal places). As in other similar calculations, to reduce any error caused by decimal places the fraction was left as '80÷60' rather than '1.33' in the last calculation.

Therefore, to the nearest drop, we need to set the giving set to 13 drops per minute to provide a dose of 800 mg/hour of drug if the solution in the infusion bag is 10 mg/mL.

---

## Questions section 6

If you could not answer or got the wrong answer for any of the questions within section 6, we suggest that you revisit the contents of Chapter 7. Specifically:

- Diagnostic Test 2—Question 28—see section 7.2.1.
- Diagnostic Test 2—Question 29—see section 7.2.1.
- Diagnostic Test 2—Question 30—see section 7.3.
- Diagnostic Test 2—Question 31—see section 7.4.
- Diagnostic Test 2—Question 32—see section 7.5.2.

**FEEDBACK**

## Diagnostic calculations test 2

### Section 7

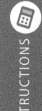

## The use of calculators for the diagnostic assessment questions in section 7

It is recommended that you undertake the calculations in section 7 using a calculator.

**INSTRUCTIONS**

**QUESTION 33:** *The following equations each represent a straight-line plot on a graph. From the equations, identify the gradient and the y intercept for each.*

    *a)* $y = 27x - 5.3$.

    *b)* $y = 0.12x$.

    *c)* $\ln[H^+] = -2.303pH$ *(where $\ln[H^+]$ is plotted against pH)*.

    *d)* $\ln(y) = 2.06 - 0.31x$.

**ANSWER:**

    a) Gradient is 27, y intercept is −5.3.

    b) Gradient is 0.12, y intercept is 0.

    c) Gradient is −2.303, y intercept is 0.

    d) Gradient is −0.31, y intercept is 2.06.

**QUESTION 34:** *Log linearize the following functions:*

    *a)* $y = 100x^{-7}$.

    *b)* $y = e^{-2x}$.

    *c)* $y = 3^x$.

    *d)* $C_t = 6e^{-5t}$.

ANSWER:     a) $\log(y) = 2 - 7\log(x)$.

b) $\ln(y) = -2x$.

c) $\log(y) = 0.48x$.

d) $\ln C_t = 1.79 - 5t$.

---

**QUESTION 35:**  *A drug is shown to degrade by first order rate kinetics. If the rate constant $k_1 = 0.004\ day^{-1}$, what percentage of drug will remain after 15 days?*

ANSWER:     $\ln C_t = \ln C_0 - k.t.$

$\ln C_t = \ln 100 - 0.004*15$.

$\ln C_t = 4.61 - 0.06 = 4.55$.

$C_t = 94\%$ of the drug will be remaining after 15 days.

---

**QUESTION 36:**  *In the above example, calculate the overage required to ensure a drug concentration of 95 mg/mL after 30 days.*

ANSWER:     In this instance we know we want $C_t = 95$ mg/mL after 30 days, so we need to identify what the starting concentration ($C_0$) should be.

$\ln C_t = \ln C_0 - k.t.$

$\ln(95) = \ln C_0 - 0.004*30$.

$\ln C_0 = 4.55 + 0.12 = 4.67$.

$C_0 = 107$ mg/mL.

---

**QUESTION 37:**  *Consider the following results in the comparison of a new drug and placebo in the reduction of blood pressure in a study. Use the 95% confidence intervals to determine if the differences seen are significant.*

|                          | % Number of cases of reduced blood pressure (95% CI) |
| ------------------------ | --------------------------------------------------- |
| Group receiving new drug | 8.8% (8.0–9.1)                                      |
| Placebo group            | 7.1% (6.2–7.7)                                      |

ANSWER:     In this study the confidence intervals do not overlap, suggesting these results are significantly different.

---

## Questions section 7

If you could not answer or got the wrong answer for any of the questions within section 7, we suggest that you revisit the contents of Chapter 8. Specifically:

- Diagnostic Test 2—Question 33—see section 8.3.1.
- Diagnostic Test 2—Question 34—see section 8.3.2.
- Diagnostic Test 2—Question 35—see section 8.4.
- Diagnostic Test 2—Question 36—see section 8.4.1.
- Diagnostic Test 2—Question 37—see section 8.5.

FEEDBACK

# 2 Pharmaceutical mathematical terminology

## 2.1 Chapter introduction

This chapter has been designed to introduce the range of mathematical terminology used within the fields of pharmaceutical compounding and medication supply. Depending on your level of study within your course as a student pharmacist or pharmacy technician, much of this chapter may be familiar to you. However, it is possible that even for individuals who have been studying pharmacy for a number of years, parts of this chapter may be unfamiliar or contain material which you may want to revisit. Owing to the risk caused by incorrect calculation of a pharmaceutical dose because of unfamiliarity with one or more pharmaceutical terms, it is vital that you are confident you understand the contents of this chapter and can easily interpret pharmaceutical terminology without error.

## 2.2 Converting between standard units

In essence, there are two basic types of conversion between standard units with which you need to become familiar. These are (a) conversion between units within the same system, just at a differing magnitude, and (b) conversion between units of different systems; both will be covered within this chapter, the first within this section and the second within section 2.5.

Calculations involving conversions between units within the same system involve alteration of a particular value from one magnitude to another. For example, the conversion of a patient's dose from milligrams (mg) to grams (g). Before we encounter these calculations, it is important to understand (i) the primary units used within pharmaceutical compounding, and (ii) the recognized abbreviations attached to these units.

In moving between units, it is important to remember the following general principles:

- Wherever possible, avoid the use of excessive zeros. The addition of unnecessary zeros can lead to confusion if read quickly or written unclearly. For example, 5 L (five litres) if written 5.0 L could, if read quickly or written unclearly be misinterpreted as 50 L (fifty litres).

- Ideally, values should be expressed in the most sensible unit to allow a reduction in the use of unnecessary zeros. Within this section of the chapter, you will be asked to convert between units and give values which include a number of zeros; this is to ensure that you are comfortable with the concept of changing between units. In standard pharmaceutical practice, it is important to try and minimize the use of unnecessary zeros whenever possible to avoid dosing errors. For example, 0.001 g would be better written as 1 mg.

---

### The use of zeros

Whenever possible, the use of excessive zeros should be avoided to minimize the risk of medication dosing error which could occur as a result of misinterpretation. Specifically:

- Whole integers should not be written with any decimal places (for example, '7 mg' not '7.0 mg').
- Units of the appropriate magnitude should be used whenever possible to avoid the inclusion of unnecessary zeros (for example, '7 mg' not '0.007 g' or '7000 micrograms').

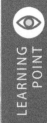

LEARNING POINT

---

## 2.2.1 Weight

The standard unit used within pharmaceutical compounding relating to weight (either the weight of a pharmaceutical ingredient or the weight of a patient) is the gram. This is abbreviated to 'g'. Moving up or down in multiples of 1000 provides the different scales used. These are summarized, along with the acceptable pharmaceutical abbreviations in Table 2.1.

---

### Abbreviations for micrograms and nanograms

Microgram and nanogram are always written in full. The abbreviations 'mcg' or 'µg', and 'ng' could all be mistaken for 'mg' (i.e. milligram), especially when handwritten, leading to a potential dosing error.

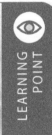

LEARNING POINT

---

It is vitally important that you familiarize yourself with the manipulation of different weights between the differing units. Failure to master this technique will potentially result in large dosing errors and the likelihood of placing the patient at risk.

| Unit | Relationship to the gram | Approved abbreviation | Equivalent scientific unit |
|---|---|---|---|
| **1 kilogram** | 1000 g | 1 kg | $1 \times 10^3$ |
| **1 gram** | 1 g | 1 g | 1 |
| **1 milligram** | 0.001 g | 1 mg | $1 \times 10^{-3}$ |
| **1 microgram** | 0.000 001 g | 1 microgram | $1 \times 10^{-6}$ |
| **1 nanogram** | 0.000 000 001 g | 1 nanogram | $1 \times 10^{-9}$ |

**Table 2.1** Standard units for weight commonly used in pharmaceutical compounding

| EXAMPLE 2:1 | |
|---|---|
| **Question:** | What is 0.1 g in milligrams, micrograms, and nanograms? |
| **Answer:** | This calculation involves moving down the weight units (as outlined in Table 2.1) in multiples of 1000. Therefore: |
| | 0.1 g in milligrams = 0.1 × 1000 = 100 mg. |
| | Continuing down the weight units, we can move from milligrams to micrograms by multiplying by another 1000. |
| | 100 mg (0.1 g) in micrograms = 100 × 1000 = 100 000 micrograms. |
| | Continuing down the weight units, we can move from micrograms to nanograms by multiplying by another 1000. |
| | 100 000 micrograms (100 mg; 0.1 g) in nanograms = 100 000 × 1000 = 100 000 000 nanograms. |

| EXAMPLE 2:2 | |
|---|---|
| **Question:** | What is 0.25 g in nanograms? |
| **Answer:** | This calculation involves moving down the weight units (as outlined in Table 2.1) in multiples of 1000. However, in this case, the question asks for the answer in nanograms, without reporting the intermediate units (i.e. the milligrams and the micrograms). Rather than moving straight from grams to nanograms, it is suggested that you attempt the question in stages, moving through the intermediary units. Therefore: |
| | 0.25 g in milligrams = 0.25 × 1000 = 250 mg. |
| | Continuing down the weight units, we can move from milligrams to micrograms by multiplying by another 1000. |
| | 250 mg (0.25 g) in micrograms = 250 × 1000 = 250 000 micrograms. |
| | Continuing down the weight units, we can move from micrograms to nanograms by multiplying by another 1000. |
| | 250 000 micrograms (250 mg; 0.25 g) in nanograms = 250 000 × 1000 = 250 000 000 nanograms. |

| EXAMPLE 2:3 | |
|---|---|
| **Question:** | What are 1050 nanograms in micrograms and milligrams? |
| **Answer:** | This calculation involves moving up the weight units (as outlined in Table 2.1) in multiples of 1000. Therefore: |
| | 1050 nanograms in micrograms = 1050 ÷ 1000 = 1.05 micrograms. |
| | Continuing up the weight units, we can move from micrograms to milligrams by dividing by another 1000. |
| | 1.05 micrograms (1050 nanograms) in milligrams = 1.05 ÷ 1000 = 0.00105 milligrams. |

## 2.2.2 Volume

The standard unit used within pharmaceutical compounding relating to volume (either the volume of a pharmaceutical ingredient or the volume of distribution of a drug within a patient) is the litre. This is abbreviated to 'L'. Moving up or down in multiples of 1000 provides the different scales used. These are summarized, along with the acceptable pharmaceutical abbreviations in Table 2.2.

| Unit | Relationship to the litre | Approved abbreviation | Equivalent scientific unit |
|------|---------------------------|-----------------------|----------------------------|
| 1 litre | 1 L | 1 L | 1 |
| 1 millilitre | 0.001 L | 1 mL | $1 \times 10^{-3}$ |
| 1 microlitre | 0.000 001 L | 1 microlitre | $1 \times 10^{-6}$ |
| 1 nanolitre | 0.000 000 001 L | 1 nanolitre | $1 \times 10^{-9}$ |

**Table 2.2** Standard units for volume commonly used in pharmaceutical compounding

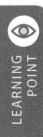

### Abbreviations for microlitre and nanolitre

Microlitre and nanolitre are always written in full. The abbreviations 'mcL' or 'µL', and 'nL' could all be mistaken for 'mL' (i.e. millilitre), especially when handwritten, leading to a potential dosing error.

LEARNING POINT

| | EXAMPLE 2:4 |
|---|---|
| **Question:** | What is 0.1 L in millilitres, microlitres, and nanolitres? |
| **Answer:** | This calculation involves moving down the volume units (as outlined in Table 2.2) in multiples of 1000. Therefore: |
| | 0.1 L in millilitres $= 0.1 \times 1000 = 100$ mL. |
| | Continuing down the volume units, we can move from millilitres to microlitres by multiplying by another 1000. |
| | 100 mL (0.1 L) in microlitres $= 100 \times 1000 = 100\,000$ microlitres. |
| | Continuing down the volume units, we can move from microlitres to nanolitres by multiplying by another 1000. |
| | 100 000 microlitres (100 mL; 0.1 L) in nanolitres $= 100\,000 \times 1000 = 100\,000\,000$ nanolitres. |

| EXAMPLE 2:5 | |
| --- | --- |
| **Question:** | What is 0.56 L in nanolitres? |
| **Answer:** | This calculation involves moving down the volume units (as outlined in Table 2.2) in multiples of 1000. However, in this case, the question asks for the answer in nanolitres, without reporting the intermediate units (i.e. the millilitres and the microlitres). Rather than moving straight from litres to nanolitres, it is suggested that you attempt the question in stages, moving through the intermediary units. Therefore: |

$$0.56\,L \text{ in millilitres} = 0.56 \times 1000 = 560\,mL.$$

Continuing down the volume units, we can move from millilitres to microlitres by multiplying by another 1000.

$$560\,mL\,(0.56\,L) \text{ in microlitres} = 560 \times 1000 = 560\,000 \text{ microlitres.}$$

Continuing down the volume units, we can move from microlitres to nanolitres by multiplying by another 1000.

$$560\,000 \text{ microlitres } (560\,mL; 0.56\,L) \text{ in nanolitres}$$
$$= 560\,000 \times 1000 = 560\,000\,000 \text{ nanolitres.}$$

| EXAMPLE 2:6 | |
| --- | --- |
| **Question:** | What is 2346 nanolitres in microlitres and millilitres? |
| **Answer:** | This calculation involves moving up the volume units (as outlined in Table 2.2) in multiples of 1000. Therefore: |

$$2346 \text{ nanolitres in microlitres} = 2346 \div 1000 = 2.346 \text{ microlitres.}$$

Continuing up the volume units, we can move from microlitres to millilitres by dividing by another 1000.

$$2.346 \text{ micrograms (2346 nanolitres) in millilitres}$$
$$= 2.346 \div 1000 = 0.002\,346 \text{ millilitres.}$$

## 2.3 Specific pharmaceutical mathematical terminology

Modern pharmaceutical practice relies on individuals understanding a number of specific abbreviations. Without this knowledge, you will find many of the calculations described within this book difficult. This section will highlight the core pharmaceutical mathematical terminology used in modern practice and it is expected that you will become familiar with these terms and understand their use before attempting some of the other sections of this book.

### 2.3.1 Percentages

Calculations involving percentages will be discussed in much more detail in Chapter 6 (see section 6.2). However, the basic terminology involved with percentages will be covered here. The term 'per cent' is often used when describing the concentration of an active ingredient within a pharmaceutical preparation without any additional qualification.

For example, 'the cream contained 2% of active ingredient'. Without any additional qualification it is necessary to understand to what the percentage is referring.

Essentially, there are two categories of active ingredients included in pharmaceutical preparations: solids and liquids. Some pharmaceutical preparations involve the use of gases but these are reasonably specialized and beyond the remit of this book.

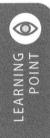

**The term 'percentage' refers to:**

the amount of solid in grams (g) or the amount of liquid in millilitres (mL) in 100 grams (g) of solid or 100 millilitres (mL) of liquid.

LEARNING POINT

A summary of the terms used can be found in Table 2.3.

| Term | Meaning | Example |
|---|---|---|
| % w/w (percentage weight in weight) | Amount of solid in grams in 100 grams of pharmaceutical product | 10% w/w = 10 g of active ingredient in every 100 g of pharmaceutical product |
| % w/v (percentage weight in volume) | Amount of solid in grams in 100 millilitres of pharmaceutical product | 10% w/v = 10 g of active ingredient in every 100 mL of pharmaceutical product |
| % v/v (percentage volume in volume) | Amount of liquid in millilitres in 100 millilitres of pharmaceutical product | 10% v/v = 10 mL of active ingredient in every 100 mL of pharmaceutical product |
| % v/w (percentage volume in weight) | Amount of liquid in millilitres in 100 grams of pharmaceutical product | 10% v/w = 10 mL of active ingredient in every 100 g of pharmaceutical product |

**Table 2.3**  A summary of the percentage terms commonly encountered in pharmaceutical practice

| | **EXAMPLE 2:7** |
|---|---|
| **Question:** | A cream contains 2% w/w of active ingredient. How much active ingredient would be present in 60 g of cream? |
| **Answer:** | If the cream contains 2% w/w of active ingredient, this means that there are 2 g of active ingredient in every 100 g of product. Therefore, in 60 g there would be:<br><br>$(2 \div 100) \times 60 = 1.2 \, g.$<br><br>Therefore, there is 1.2 g of active ingredient in 60 g of the cream. |

| **EXAMPLE 2:8** | |
|---|---|
| **Question:** | You are asked to make 250 mL pharmaceutical product which contains 0.25% w/v of an active ingredient. How much active ingredient is required? |
| **Answer:** | If the final pharmaceutical product contains 0.25% w/v, this means that there is 0.25 g (or 250 mg) in every 100 mL of the product. Therefore, in 250 mL of product, there would be:<br><br>$$(0.25 \div 100) \times 250 = 0.625 \, \text{g} \equiv 625 \, \text{mg}.$$<br><br>Therefore, you will need 625 mg of active ingredient to make 250 mL of a 0.25% w/v pharmaceutical product. Note that the answer has been expressed as 625 mg, rather than 0.625 g to avoid the use of both a leading zero and a decimal which could, when written down, easily be mistaken for an alternative quantity. |

| **EXAMPLE 2:9** | |
|---|---|
| **Question:** | How much active ingredient is present in 350 g of a 3% v/w ointment? |
| **Answer:** | If the final pharmaceutical product contains 3% v/w, this means that there are 3 mL in every 100 g of the product. Therefore, in 350 g of product, there would be:<br><br>$$(3 \div 100) \times 350 = 10.5 \, \text{mL}.$$<br><br>Therefore, there are 10.5 mL of active ingredient in 350 g of the cream. |

### 2.3.2 Solubility

More complex calculations involving solubility will be covered in Chapter 6 (see section 6.3 and section 6.4). However, as with percentages (see previous section) there is specific terminology relating to solubility with which you need to be familiar before tackling calculations involving solubility values.

Solubility is often expressed as '1 in x'. This (x) refers to the amount of solvent required to dissolve 1 g (or 1 mL) of ingredient.

**The terms 'solute', 'solvent', and 'solution'**

You are expected to be familiar with the following terms:

- Solute—the substance dissolved in a solvent.
- Solvent—the liquid in which a solute is dissolved.
- Solution—the resultant liquid after dissolution of a solute in a solvent. The mixture will be homogenous, that is the concentration of the solution will be the same in all parts.

LEARNING POINT

Therefore, a solubility value of, for example, 1 in 20 means that you would require 20 mL of solvent in which to dissolve every 1 g of solute. The solubility value for a particular ingredient will vary depending on the solvent being used. For example, the solubility of sodium bicarbonate in water is 1 in 12; however, it is practically insoluble in alcohol.[3]

3 *Martindale: The Complete Drug Reference*, accessed via Medicines Complete, 29 December 2012.

| | **EXAMPLE 2:10** |
|---|---|
| **Question:** | How much water would be required to dissolve 3.5 g of an ingredient which is soluble 1 in 7? |
| **Answer:** | If the ingredient is soluble 1 in 7, this means that for every 1 g of the ingredient, you require 7 mL of water. Therefore, for 3.5 g of ingredient you require:<br><br>$(7 \div 1) \times 3.5 = 24.5 \text{ mL}.$<br><br>Therefore, you will require a minimum of 24.5 mL of water to dissolve 3.5 g of an ingredient which is soluble 1 in 7 (in water). |

| | **EXAMPLE 2:11** |
|---|---|
| **Question:** | To the nearest whole number of grams, what is the maximum amount of a solute which can be dissolved in 100 mL of water if the solubility of the solute in water is 1 in 9? |
| **Answer:** | If the ingredient is soluble 1 in 9, this means that for every 1 g of the ingredient, you require 9 mL of water. Therefore, for 2 g of ingredient you require 18 mL, etc. Therefore, in 100 mL, you would be able to dissolve:<br><br>$(100 \div 9) = 11.11 \text{ g}$ (to two decimal places).<br><br>Therefore, to the nearest whole number of grams, the maximum amount of solute which can be dissolved in 100 mL of water (if the solubility of the solute in water is 1 in 9) is 11 g. |

## 2.3.3 Parts

Another method for the expression of the amount of different ingredients within a pharmaceutical preparation is to use the term 'parts'. This refers to the proportion of an ingredient in relation to the amount of other ingredients within a preparation.

| | **EXAMPLE 2:12** |
|---|---|
| **Question:** | You are required to make 350 g of a dusting powder according to the following formula:<br><br>• Ingredient A   4 parts.<br>• Ingredient B   6 parts.<br>• Ingredient C   to 20 parts.<br><br>What is the weight of each of the powders in the final preparation? |
| **Answer:** | The formula indicates that for every 20 parts of preparation, Ingredient A accounts for 4 parts and Ingredient B accounts for 6 parts. Therefore, Ingredient C accounts for:<br><br>$20 - (4 + 6) = 10 \text{ parts}.$ |

Therefore the formula for the amount of each ingredient would be the total weight of the dusting powder (350 g) divided by the total number of parts (20), then multiplied by the number of parts of that ingredient (Ingredient A, 4 parts; Ingredient B, 6 parts; Ingredient C, 10 parts).

This means that in 350 g of the dusting powder, there are the following amounts of each ingredient:

- Ingredient A    $(350 \div 20) \times 4 = 70$ g.
- Ingredient B    $(350 \div 20) \times 6 = 105$ g.
- Ingredient C    $(350 \div 20) \times 10 = 175$ g.

To check this calculation, add up the amounts of the individual ingredients and check that they total 350 g.

$70 + 105 + 175 = 350$ g.

### 2.3.4 Proportions

Another method for the expression of the amount of an ingredient or ingredients within a pharmaceutical preparation is to express the amount of ingredient to be added in relation to the amount of the vehicle or portion of the vehicle to which the ingredient is being added (e.g. to dissolve into to form a solution or to suspend within to make a suspension).

**LEARNING POINT**

**The term 'vehicle'**

The term 'vehicle' refers to the part of a pharmaceutical preparation used to deliver the active ingredients. For example, in a solution, the vehicle would be the solvent that the solute or solutes are dissolved within to form the solution. In a suspension, the solid particles are suspended throughout the liquid vehicle.

- This is why a suspension will need shaking before an accurate dose can be measured, to ensure that the active ingredient is evenly distributed throughout the vehicle before the dose is measured. With a solution, it is not necessary to shake the preparation before measuring a dose as the active ingredient is evenly distributed throughout the vehicle as the product will be a homogenous mixture.

The vehicle does not need to be a liquid; solid or semi-solid vehicles will be used in certain pharmaceutical preparations such as ointments.

The two different expressions used are as follows:

- 'to', as in '1 to 10'.
  - This expression is used to explain the number of parts (in this example, 1) which are put with the number of parts of the vehicle (in this example, 10). Therefore, for every 11 parts, one part will be ingredient and 10 will be vehicle.

- 'in', as in '1 in 10'.
  - This expression is used to explain the number of parts (in this example, 1) which are put with the total number of parts of the final product (for example, solution or suspension; in this case, 10). Therefore, for every 10 parts, one part will be ingredient and nine will be vehicle.

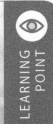

**The pharmaceutical mathematical terms 'in' and 'to'**

Remember that there is an important difference between 'in' and 'to' when used in relation to the proportion of an ingredient to be added to a pharmaceutical preparation.

- 'to' refers to the number of parts of ingredient in proportion to the number of parts of vehicle.
- 'in' refers to the number of parts of ingredient in proportion to the number of parts of final product.

Although for small amounts of active ingredient within a vehicle, the difference between the two may be negligible, as the proportion of active ingredient increases, the difference between the two becomes more marked.

LEARNING POINT

## 2.4 Interpreting dosage instructions

In addition to understanding the amount of active ingredient which is within or is to be added to a pharmaceutical preparation, it is also necessary to understand how much and how frequently a patient is required to take or use a medicinal product. Nowadays, with the predominance of computer-generated prescription forms, medication directions are much clearer and use fewer abbreviations than when prescription forms were all written by hand. Nevertheless, abbreviations are still used and it is important that you are aware of their meanings.

### 2.4.1 Abbreviations relating to the quantity to administer

In many cases, the number of dosage units or quantity of liquid medication to be administered at each point is clearly stated on the patient's prescription form; for example, 'Take TWO tablets twice a day'. It is clear from this statement that at each administration point, two dosage forms (in this case tablets) are to be taken. The same would be the case for liquid preparations, for example, 'Take TWO 5 mL spoonfuls three times a day'. As with the previous example, it is clear from this statement that the patient is to administer 10 mL (i.e. two 5 mL spoonfuls) of the liquid preparation at each administration point.

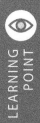

## Expressing dosage instructions

*'Take TWO tablets twice a day'.*

Note that with this dosage instruction, it has been written in a specific way to reduce the potential for misinterpretation.

- Firstly, any reference to numbers is in words.

- Secondly, the number relating to the number of dosage units to be administered at each point and the number relating to the frequency of administration have been separated by the dosage form.

If this was not the case, it could read something like: *'Take 2 2 times a day'* and be misinterpreted as 'take 22 each day'.

*'Take TWO 5 mL spoonfuls three times a day'.*

Note that as with the dosage instruction relating to solid dosage forms above, this dosage instruction has also been written in a specific way to reduce the potential for misinterpretation.

- Firstly, all references to numbers are in words except for reference to the 5 mL spoon. Wherever possible (and it is not always the case that it is), dosage instructions should avoid the use of numbers in digit format except for references to 5 mL spoons.

- Secondly, as with the solid dosage form example, the number relating to the number of 5 mL spoonfuls to be administered at each point and the number relating to the frequency of administration, have been separated by the dosage form.

However, although not recommended (owing to the potential for misinterpretation and thereby dosing error), abbreviations are sometimes encountered relating to the number of dosage units. Examples of abbreviations you may encounter are given in Figure 2.1.

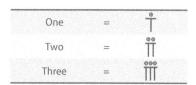

| One | = | ☓ |
| Two | = | ☓ |
| Three | = | ☓ |

**Figure 2.1** Common abbreviations for quantities of solid dosage forms to administer.

## 2.4.2 Abbreviations relating to administration frequency

In addition to the abbreviations relating to the quantities of solid dosage forms to administer, abbreviations are also used which relate to the administration frequency. Many of these are based on Latin phrases and although it is not important that you learn the Latin phrases, it is important that you are familiar with the meanings. A more comprehensive list of these abbreviations can be found in the Appendix; however, an example of some of the more common ones can be found in Table 2.4.

| Once a day | = | OD | Omni die |
|---|---|---|---|
| Twice a day | = | BD | Bis in die |
| Three times a day | = | TDS | Ter die sumendum |
| Four times a day | = | QDS | Quarter die sumendum |
| Every morning | = | OM | Omni mane |
| Every evening | = | ON | Omni nocte |

**Table 2.4** Examples of common abbreviations for frequencies of administration

# 2.5 Imperial and metric conversions

This section will explain the conversion of major units between imperial and metric systems. In addition to the need for you to be able to convert accurately between units within the same system (see section 2.2), it is also necessary at times to be able to convert values from one system to another. The primary time at which this is required within modern pharmacy practice is in conversion of a patient's weight from imperial to metric, or vice versa.

## 2.5.1 Imperial units

Before examining the methodology behind the conversion, it is necessary to recap the imperial system of weight, which uses ounces, pounds, and stones. The key units encountered in modern pharmaceutical practice are detailed in Table 2.5, including examples of the common abbreviations in use.

| 16 ounces (16 oz) | = | 1 pound (1 lb) |
|---|---|---|
| 14 pounds (14 lb) | = | 1 stone (1 st) |

**Table 2.5** Imperial system of weight

## 2.5.2 Converting weight from imperial to metric

Usually, conversion between the two systems uses a conversion factor and as such, is an approximation of the actual value rather than an absolute. However for most uses, this is sufficiently accurate.

| | **EXAMPLE 2:13** |
|---|---|
| **Question:** | A patient weighs 12 st and 8 lb and is prescribed a dose of Drug D at 2 mg/kg twice a day. What dosage should be supplied (noting that 2.2 pounds ≈ 1 kg)? |
| **Answer:** | To undertake the dosage calculation, it is first necessary to convert the patient's weight from imperial to metric. To do this, we can use the approximate conversion factor that 2.2 pounds ≈ 1 kg. |

Therefore, if 2.2 lb = 1 kg, we need to know the patient's weight in pounds. Referring to Table 2.5, we can convert the patient's weight of 12 st 8 lb into pounds as follows:

$$(12 \times 14) + 8 = 176 \, lb.$$

If 2.2 lb = 1 kg, 176 lb is the same as:

$$176 \div 2.2 = 80 \, kg.$$

Then we can use the dosage instructions of 2 mg/kg to work out the patient's dose:

$$80 \times 2 = 160 \, mg \text{ for each dose (in this case, twice a day).}$$

### 2.5.3 Converting weight from metric to imperial

| | **EXAMPLE 2:14** |
|---|---|
| **Question:** | A patient has been advised to lose 5 kg and wants to know what weight this is in pounds (noting that 2.2 pounds ≈ 1 kg). |
| **Answer:** | For this calculation, we need to multiply the number of kilograms by the conversion factor to obtain the number of pounds to advise the patient to lose. $$5 \times 2.2 = 11 \, lb.$$ Therefore, you need to advise the patient that 5 kg is (approximately) the same as 11 pounds. |

# 2.6 Self-assessment questions

## 2.6.1 Basic self-assessment questions

This section contains a number of basic self-assessment questions for you to undertake to ensure you have an understanding of the material in this chapter. It is recommended that you undertake all of these calculations **without a calculator** and then check your answers with the answers in section 2.8.

**INSTRUCTIONS**

### The use of calculators for the self-assessment questions in this chapter

It is recommended that you undertake the following calculations without the use of a calculator.

All of the self-assessment questions within this section can be undertaken using a pen and paper.

**QUESTION 2.1:**    *What is 0.45 g in milligrams, micrograms, and nanograms?*

**QUESTION 2.2:**    *What is 0.578 g in nanograms?*

**QUESTION 2.3:**    *What is 2345 nanograms in micrograms and milligrams?*

**QUESTION 2.4:**    *What is 0.75 L in millilitres, microlitres, and nanolitres?*

**QUESTION 2.5:**    *What is 0.96 L in nanolitres?*

**QUESTION 2.6:**    *What is 1500 nanolitres in microlitres and millilitres?*

**QUESTION 2.7:**    *A cream contains 3.5% w/w of active ingredient. How much active ingredient would be present in 150 g of cream?*

**QUESTION 2.8:**    *A cream contains 15% w/w of active ingredient. How much active ingredient would be present in 500 g of cream?*

**QUESTION 2.9:**    *You are asked to make 300 mL pharmaceutical product which contains 0.45% w/v of an active ingredient. How much active ingredient is required?*

**QUESTION 2.10:**    *You are asked to make 750 mL pharmaceutical product which contains 3.25% w/v of an active ingredient. How much active ingredient is required?*

**QUESTION 2.11:**    *How much active ingredient is present in 650 g of a 7.5% v/w ointment?*

**QUESTION 2.12:**    *How much active ingredient is present in 1000 mL of a 45% v/v solution?*

**QUESTION 2.13:**    *How much water would be required to dissolve 15.6 g of an ingredient which is soluble 1 in 14?*

**QUESTION 2.14:**    *To the nearest whole number of grams, what is the maximum amount of a solute which can be dissolved in 350 mL of water if the solubility of the solute in water is 1 in 6?*

**QUESTION 2.15:**    *You are required to make 550 g of a dusting powder according to the following formula:*

- *Ingredient A    3 parts.*
- *Ingredient B    8 parts.*
- *Ingredient C    to 20 parts.*

*What is the weight of each of the powders in the final preparation?*

**QUESTION 2.16:**    *How much of a liquid ingredient is required for 900 mL of a 1 in 20 solution?*

**QUESTION 2.17:**    *How much of a liquid ingredient is required for 900 mL of a 1 to 20 solution?*

**QUESTION 2.18:**    *A patient weighs 9 st and 10 lb and is prescribed a dose of Drug E at 4.5 mg/kg once a day. What dosage should be supplied? (Note: there are approximately 2.2 pounds in a kilogram.)*

**QUESTION 2.19:**    *A patient has been advised to lose 7.5 kg and wants to know what weight this is in pounds. (Note: there are approximately 2.2 pounds in a kilogram.)*

### 2.6.2 Running case studies

**QUESTION 2.20:**

*Evie Jones has been prescribed a cream which contains 2.5% w/w active ingredient. It is advised that for a patient of her age, no more than 5 g of active ingredient is applied in any 1-week period.*

*Mary Jones is worried that she may be applying too much cream and asks what is the maximum amount of cream that could be applied in a week? The cream comes in 50 g tubes.*

**QUESTION 2.21:**

*Bob has been prescribed a concentrated foot soak which he needs to dilute before use. The instruction Bob has been provided with says that he is to dilute '1 in 25' and use around 1 L of soak at each time. Bob is unsure how much of the concentrated foot soak to use and how to dilute it and asks you for advice.*

**QUESTION 2.22:**

*John Jones has been told that in addition to giving up smoking, he would be advised to keep an eye on his weight. He is told that in relation to his height, his current weight is fine. John wants to know what his weight is in stones and pounds so he can keep an eye on it. What is John's weight in stones and pounds? (Note: there are approximately 2.2 pounds in a kilogram.)*

**QUESTION 2.23:**

*To register at the local childminder, Mary and John Jones have to fill in a form about George. They are asked to complete this with George's weight in stones and pounds and ask if you can help. What is George's weight in stones and pounds? (Note: there are approximately 2.2 pounds in a kilogram.)*

**QUESTION 2.24:**

*Geoff has been told to make sure his weight does not go over 85 kg. He only understands imperial weights for body weight and so asks you what he currently weighs in kilograms and what the imperial equivalent of 85 kg would be? (Note: there are approximately 2.2 pounds in a kilogram.)*

## 2.7 Summary

This chapter has summarized the key terminology with which you need to be familiar to tackle the core chapters within this book. Some of the material presented within this chapter may have been familiar to you; however, it is in the interpretation of common pharmaceutical mathematical scenarios, or, more importantly, the misinterpretation of the pharmaceutical mathematical terminology contained within the scenarios, where simple but potentially damaging mistakes can occur. It is expected that you are familiar with the terminology covered within this chapter before tackling the remaining chapters.

## 2.8 Answers to self-assessment questions

This section contains the worked answers for the self-assessment questions within section 2.6.

**The use of calculators for the self-assessment questions in this chapter**

It is recommended that you undertake the following calculations without the use of a calculator.

All of the self-assessment questions within this section can be undertaken using a pen and paper.

INSTRUCTIONS

---

**QUESTION 2.1:**   *What is 0.45 g in milligrams, micrograms, and nanograms?*

**ANSWER:**   This calculation involves moving down the weight units (as outlined in Table 2.1) in multiples of 1000. Therefore:

0.45 g in milligrams = 0.45 × 1000 = 450 mg.

Continuing down the weight units, we can move from milligrams to micrograms by multiplying by another 1000.

450 mg (0.45 g) in micrograms = 450 × 1000 = 450 000 micrograms.

Continuing down the weight units, we can move from micrograms to nanograms by multiplying by another 1000.

450 000 micrograms (450 mg; 0.45 g) in nanograms
= 450 000 × 1000 = 450 000 000 nanograms.

---

**QUESTION 2.2:**   *What is 0.578 g in nanograms?*

**ANSWER:**   This calculation involves moving down the weight units (as outlined in Table 2.1) in multiples of 1000. However, in this case, the question asks for the answer in nanograms, without reporting the intermediate units (i.e. the milligrams and the micrograms). Rather than moving straight from grams to nanograms, it is suggested that you attempt the question in stages, moving through the intermediary units. Therefore:

0.578 g in milligrams = 0.578 × 1000 = 578 mg.

Continuing down the weight units, we can move from milligrams to micrograms by multiplying by another 1000.

578 mg (0.578 g) in micrograms = 578 × 1000 = 578 000 micrograms.

Continuing down the weight units, we can move from micrograms to nanograms by multiplying by another 1000.

578 000 micrograms (578 mg; 0.578 g) in nanograms
= 578 000 × 1000 = 578 000 000 nanograms.

| QUESTION 2.3: | *What is 2345 nanograms in micrograms and milligrams?* |
|---|---|
| ANSWER: | This calculation involves moving up the weight units (as outlined in Table 2.1) in multiples of 1000. Therefore: |

2345 nanograms in micrograms = 2345 ÷ 1000 = 2.345 micrograms.

Continuing up the weight units, we can move from milligrams to micrograms by dividing by another 1000.

2.345 micrograms (2345 nanograms) in milligrams
= 2.345 ÷ 1000 = 0.002 345 milligrams.

| QUESTION 2.4: | *What is 0.75 L in millilitres, microlitres, and nanolitres?* |
|---|---|
| ANSWER: | This calculation involves moving down the volume units (as outlined in Table 2.2) in multiples of 1000. Therefore: |

0.75 L in millilitres = 0.75 × 1000 = 750 mL.

Continuing down the volume units, we can move from millilitres to microlitres by multiplying by another 1000.

750 mL (0.75 L) in microlitres = 750 × 1000 = 750 000 microlitres.

Continuing down the volume units, we can move from microlitres to nanolitres by multiplying by another 1000.

750 000 microlitres (750 mL; 0.75 L) in nanolitres
= 750 000 × 1000 = 750 000 000 nanolitres.

| QUESTION 2.5: | *What is 0.96 L in nanolitres?* |
|---|---|
| ANSWER: | This calculation involves moving down the volume units (as outlined in Table 2.2) in multiples of 1000. However, in this case, the question asks for the answer in nanolitres, without reporting the intermediate units (i.e. the millilitres and the microlitres). Rather than moving straight from litres to nanolitres, it is suggested that you attempt the question in stages, moving through the intermediary units. Therefore: |

0.96 L in millilitres = 0.96 × 1000 = 960 mL.

Continuing down the volume units, we can move from millilitres to microlitres by multiplying by another 1000.

960 mL (0.96 L) in microlitres = 960 × 1000 = 960 000 microlitres.

Continuing down the volume units, we can move from microlitres to nanolitres by multiplying by another 1000.

960 000 microlitres (960 mL; 0.96 L) in nanolitres
= 960 000 × 1000 = 960 000 000 nanolitres.

**QUESTION 2.6:** *What is 1500 nanolitres in microlitres and millilitres?*

**ANSWER:** This calculation involves moving up the volume units (as outlined in Table 2.2) in multiples of 1000. Therefore:

1500 nanolitres in microlitres = 1500 ÷ 1000 = 1.5 microlitres.

Continuing up the volume units, we can move from microlitres to millilitres by dividing by another 1000.

1.5 microlitres (1500 nanolitres) in millilitres
= 1.5 ÷ 1000 = 0.0015 millilitres.

**QUESTION 2.7:** *A cream contains 3.5% w/w of active ingredient. How much active ingredient would be present in 150 g of cream?*

**ANSWER:** If the cream contains 3.5% w/w of active ingredient, this means that there are 3.5 g in every 100 g of product. Therefore, in 150 g there would be:

(3.5 ÷ 100) × 150 = 5.25 g.

Therefore, there are 5.25 g of active ingredient in 150 g of the cream.

**QUESTION 2.8:** *A cream contains 15% w/w of active ingredient. How much active ingredient would be present in 500 g of cream?*

**ANSWER:** If the cream contains 15% w/w of active ingredient, this means that there are 15 g in every 100 g of product. Therefore, in 500 g there would be:

(15 ÷ 100) × 500 = 75 g.

Therefore, there are 75 g of active ingredient in 500 g of the cream.

**QUESTION 2.9:** *You are asked to make 300 mL pharmaceutical product which contains 0.45% w/v of an active ingredient. How much active ingredient is required?*

**ANSWER:** If the final pharmaceutical product contains 0.45% w/v, this means that there is 0.45 g (or 450 mg) in every 100 mL of the product. Therefore, in 300 mL of product, there would be:

(0.45 ÷ 100) × 300 = 1.35 g.

Therefore, you will need 1.35 g of active ingredient to make 300 mL of a 0.45% w/v pharmaceutical product.

**QUESTION 2.10:** *You are asked to make 750 mL pharmaceutical product which contains 3.25% w/v of an active ingredient. How much active ingredient is required?*

**ANSWER:** If the final pharmaceutical product contains 3.25% w/v, this means that there are 3.25 g in every 100 mL of the product. Therefore, in 750 mL of product, there would be:

(3.25 ÷ 100) × 750 = 24.375 g.

Therefore, you will need 24.375 g of active ingredient to make 750 mL of a 3.25% w/v pharmaceutical product.

**QUESTION 2.11:** *How much active ingredient is present in 650 g of a 7.5% v/w ointment?*

**ANSWER:** If the final pharmaceutical product contains 7.5% v/w, this means that there are 7.5 mL in every 100 g of the product. Therefore, in 650 g of product, there would be:

(7.5 ÷ 100) × 650 = 48.75 mL.

Therefore, there are 48.75 mL of active ingredient in 650 g of the pharmaceutical product.

**QUESTION 2.12:** *How much active ingredient is present in 1000 mL of a 45% v/v solution?*

**ANSWER:** If the final pharmaceutical product contains 45% v/v, this means that there are 45 mL in every 100 mL of the product. Therefore, in 1000 mL of product, there would be:

$$(45 \div 100) \times 1000 = 450 \, mL.$$

Therefore, there are 450 mL of active ingredient in 1000 mL of the solution.

**QUESTION 2.13:** *How much water would be required to dissolve 15.6 g of an ingredient which is soluble 1 in 14?*

**ANSWER:** If the ingredient is soluble 1 in 14, this means that for every 1 g of the ingredient, you require 14 mL of solvent. Therefore, for 15.6 g of ingredient you will require:

$$(14 \div 1) \times 15.6 = 218.4 \, mL.$$

Therefore, you will require a minimum of 218.4 mL of solvent to dissolve 15.6 g of an ingredient which is soluble 1 in 14.

**QUESTION 2.14:** *To the nearest whole number of grams, what is the maximum amount of a solute which can be dissolved in 350 mL of water if the solubility of the solute in water is 1 in 6?*

**ANSWER:** If the ingredient is soluble 1 in 6, this means that for every 1 g of the ingredient, you require 6 mL of water. Therefore, for 2 g of ingredient you will require 12 mL, etc. Therefore, in 350 mL, you would be able to dissolve:

$$(350 \div 6) = 58.33 \, g \text{ (to two decimal places).}$$

Therefore, to the nearest whole number of grams, the maximum amount of solute which can be dissolved in 350 mL of water (if the solubility of the solute in water is 1 in 6) is 58 g.

**QUESTION 2.15:** *You are required to make 550 g of a dusting powder according to the following formula:*

- *Ingredient A   3 parts.*
- *Ingredient B   8 parts.*
- *Ingredient C   to 20 parts.*

*What is the weight of each of the powders in the final preparation?*

**ANSWER:** The formula indicates that for every 20 parts of preparation, Ingredient A accounts for 3 parts and Ingredient B accounts for 8 parts. Therefore, Ingredient C accounts for:

$$20 - (3 + 8) = 9 \text{ parts.}$$

Therefore, the formula for the amount of each ingredient would be the total weight of the dusting powder (550 g) divided by the total number of parts (20), then multiplied by the number of parts of that ingredient (Ingredient A, 3 parts; Ingredient B, 8 parts; Ingredient C, 9 parts).

This means that in 550 g of the dusting powder, there are the following amounts of each ingredient:

- Ingredient A    $(550 \div 20) \times 3 = 82.5$ g.
- Ingredient B    $(550 \div 20) \times 8 = 220$ g.
- Ingredient C    $(550 \div 20) \times 9 = 247.5$ g.

To check this calculation, add up the amounts of the individual ingredients and check that they total 550 g.

$82.5 + 220 + 247.5 = 550$ g.

---

**QUESTION 2.16:**  *How much of a liquid ingredient is required for 900 mL of a 1 in 20 solution?*

**ANSWER:**  If the solute is to be added to form a 1 in 20 solution, this means that for every 20 mL of solution, 1 mL will be solute. Therefore in 900 mL, there will be:

$900 \div 20 = 45$ mL of the liquid ingredient.

Therefore, we require 45 mL of the ingredient and dissolve this in $(900 - 45) = 855$ mL of solvent.

---

**QUESTION 2.17:**  *How much of a liquid ingredient is required for 900 mL of a 1 to 20 solution?*

**ANSWER:**  If the solute is to be added to form a 1 to 20 solution, this means that for every 21 mL of solution $(20 + 1)$, 1 mL will be solute. Therefore in 900 mL, there will be:

$900 \div 21 = 42.86$ mL of the liquid ingredient (to two decimal places).

Therefore, we require 42.86 mL of the ingredient and dissolve this in $(900 - 42.86) = 857.14$ mL of solvent (both to two decimal places).

Note: compare the answers to Question 2.16 and Question 2.17. Although both use the same final volume of solution and both have '1' and '20' in the proportions, because the first uses 'in' and the second uses 'to', the answers are different.

---

**QUESTION 2.18:**  *A patient weighs 9 st and 10 lb and is prescribed a dose of Drug E at 4.5 mg/kg once a day. What dosage should be supplied? (Note: there are approximately 2.2 pounds in a kilogram.)*

**ANSWER:**  To undertake the dosage calculation, it is first necessary to convert the patient's weight from imperial to metric. To do this, we can use the approximate conversion factor that 2.2 pounds ≈ 1 kg.

Therefore, if 2.2 lb = 1 kg, we need to know the patient's weight in pounds. Referring to Table 2.5, we can convert the patient's weight of 9 st 10 lb into pounds as follows:

$(9 \times 14) + 10 = 136$ lb.

If 2.2 lb = 1 kg, 136 lb is the same as:

$136 \div 2.2 = 61.82$ kg (to two decimal places).

Then we can use the dosage instructions of 4.5 mg/kg to work out the patient's dose:

$61.82 \times 4.5 = 278$ mg (to the nearest milligram) for each dose (in this case, once a day).

**QUESTION 2.19:**    *A patient has been advised to lose 7.5 kg and wants to know what weight this is in pounds. (Note: there are approximately 2.2 pounds in a kilogram.)*

**ANSWER:**    For this calculation, we need to multiply the number of kilograms by the conversion factor (approximately 2.2 pounds in a kilogram) to obtain the number of pounds to advise the patient to lose.

$$7.5 \times 2.2 = 16.5 \, \text{lb}.$$

Therefore, you need to advise the patient that 7.5 kg is (approximately) the same as 16.5 pounds (or 1 stone and 2.5 pounds).

**QUESTION 2.20:**

*Evie Jones has been prescribed a cream which contains 2.5% w/w active ingredient. It is advised that for a patient of her age, no more than 5 g of active ingredient is applied in any 1-week period.*

*Mary Jones is worried that she may be applying too much cream and asks what is the maximum amount of cream that could be applied in a week? The cream comes in 50 g tubes.*

**ANSWER:**

If the cream contains 2.5% w/w, this means that in every 100 g, there are 2.5 g of active ingredient. Therefore, in every 50 g of cream (i.e. each tube), there are:

$$(2.5 \div 100) \times 50 = 1.25 \, \text{g}.$$

If the maximum amount of active ingredient which can be applied in a week is 5 g, this would equate to the following number of tubes:

$$5 \div 1.25 \, \text{g} = 4 \, \text{tubes}.$$

Therefore, you can advise Mary Jones that the maximum amount that can be applied to Evie in a week is four tubes of cream.

**QUESTION 2.21:**

*Bob has been prescribed a concentrated foot soak which he needs to dilute before use. The instruction Bob has been provided with says that he is to dilute '1 in 25' and use around 1 L of soak at each time. Bob is unsure how much of the concentrated foot soak to use and how to dilute it and asks you for advice.*

**ANSWER:**

The instruction Bob has been provided with his foot soak is to dilute '1 in 25'. This means that for every 25 parts of the final soak, one part will be the concentrated soak (i.e. 1 part concentrate with 24 parts diluent). If each soak he is to use has a total volume of 1 L, this means that Bob needs to use:

$(1 \div 25) \times 1 = 0.04\,L \equiv 40\,mL.$

Therefore, you need to advise Bob to use 40 mL of the concentrated foot soak and dilute to a final volume of 1 L. In addition, you may need to explain to Bob how he is to measure 40 mL and 1 L at home to ensure that he is able to make up the foot soak accurately.

---

**QUESTION 2.22:**

*John Jones has been told that in addition to giving up smoking, he would be advised to keep an eye on his weight. He is told that in relation to his height, his current weight is fine. John wants to know what his weight is in stones and pounds so he can keep an eye on it. What is John's weight in stones and pounds? (Note: there are approximately 2.2 pounds in a kilogram.)*

**ANSWER:**

John Jones currently weighs 80 kg. Therefore, firstly, we need to convert his weight to pounds:

$80 \times 2.2 = 176$ pounds.

Next, we need to convert this to stone and pounds. To do this we need to work out the number of whole stones within the 176 pounds. This can be achieved by dividing the number of pounds by 14.

$176 \div 14 = 12.57$ (to two decimal places).

To convert the 0.57 stone to pounds, we need to work out what this is in fourteenths (as there are 14 pounds in a stone).

$(14 \div 1) \times 0.57 = 7.98.$

Therefore, John Jones weighs 12 stone and 8 pounds (to the nearest pound).

---

**QUESTION 2.23:**

*To register at the local childminder, Mary and John Jones have to fill in a form about George. They are asked to complete this with George's weight in stones and pounds and ask if you can help. What is George's weight in stones and pounds? (Note: there are approximately 2.2 pounds in a kilogram.)*

**ANSWER:**

Currently, George weighs 13.7 kg. Therefore, firstly, we need to convert this weight to pounds:

$13.7 \times 2.2 = 30.14$ pounds.

Next, we need to convert this to stone and pounds. To do this we need to work out the number of whole stones within the 30.14 pounds. This can be achieved by dividing the number of pounds by 14.

$30.14 \div 14 = 2.15$ (to two decimal places).

To convert the 0.15 stone to pounds, we need to work out what this is in fourteenths (as there are 14 pounds in a stone).

$(14 \div 1) \times 0.15 = 2.1.$

Therefore, George weighs 2 stone and 2 pounds (to the nearest pound).

**QUESTION 2.24:**

*Geoff has been told to make sure his weight does not go over 85 kg. He only understands imperial weights for body weight and so asks you what he currently weighs in kilograms and what the imperial equivalent of 85 kg would be? (Note: there are approximately 2.2 pounds in a kilogram.)*

**ANSWER:**

You need to tackle this question in two stages. Firstly, work out what Geoff's weight is in kilograms and then convert 85 kg into stone and pounds.

Geoff currently weighs 12 stone and 6 pounds. Firstly, convert this weight into pounds:

$$(12 \times 14) + 6 = 174 \text{ pounds.}$$

Next, convert this to kilograms:

$$174 \div 2.2 = 79.09 \text{ kg (to two decimal places).}$$

Therefore, you can tell Geoff that he weighs 79 kg.

Secondly, convert 85 kg to stone and pounds to give Geoff the imperial weight he has been advised not to exceed.

$$85 \times 2.2 = 187 \text{ pounds.}$$

Next, we need to convert this to stone and pounds. To do this we need to work out the number of whole stones within the 187 pounds. This can be achieved by dividing the number of pounds by 14.

$$187 \div 14 = 13.36 \text{ (to two decimal places).}$$

To convert the 0.36 stone to pounds, we need to work out what this is in fourteenths (as there are 14 pounds in a stone).

$$(14 \div 1) \times 0.36 = 5.04.$$

Therefore, you can tell Geoff that he has been advised that he should not increase his current weight of 12 stone 6 pounds (which is 79 kg) to more than 13 stone and 5 pounds (which is 85 kg).

# Mathematical basics in pharmacy: measurements and data

# 3

## 3.1 Chapter introduction

The collection and expression of data are key requirements in pharmacy. This can include considering data collected from a single patient (e.g. vancomycin concentrations in plasma), a group of patients (e.g. liver function in patients over 60), through to considering the characteristics of a patient's medicine (e.g. drug content within a batch of tablets). In the collection of these measurements, variability and uncertainties arise. These result from the measuring instrument, the environment in which the measurement is taken, and from the operator. Therefore, this chapter first considers how variation within measurements arises and then how data sets can be summarized and variability measured.

## 3.2 Variation in measurements and experimental uncertainties

No physical quantity can be measured exactly; all measurements can only be given to within a range of uncertainty. The range of uncertainty associated with a measurement is dictated by the sensitivity/limitations of the equipment taking the measurement, the process, and the user collecting the measurement. This leads to variability in data that is described as experimental uncertainties or experimental errors. Thus, experimental uncertainties refer to the disagreement between a measurement and the true or accepted measurement. It does not refer to mistakes in experiments. Experimental uncertainties are inherent in the experimental process and come from a variety of sources. The effects that give rise to uncertainty in measurements can either be:

- Random: These arise from unnoticed variations in measurement techniques and can be associated with the operator, the instruments, and the environment. In the case of random errors, repeating the measurements gives randomly different results. Random errors can arise from, for example, the sensitivity of the measuring apparatus and fluctuations in the environment.

- Systematic: These can be related to equipment and errors from controlled variables. These are errors that do not change during the measurement. These errors produce a shift in the value measured. For example, if a balance used to weigh out material is not correctly set to zero, all subsequent measurements will be out by the same amount. Systematic errors are not random, with the same error affecting the result each time it is repeated. Therefore repeating the measurements using the same procedure will not allow you to identify systematic errors. Systematic errors may be identified by performing experiments using different processes and comparing results.

The total uncertainty of a measurement is usually a combination of systematic and random effects, and given there is always a margin of uncertainty associated with any measurement, it is important to be able to express this uncertainty.

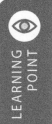

**LEARNING POINT**

### Experimental uncertainties

Physical measurements cannot be taken exactly; there is always a margin of doubt. Uncertainty is a quantification of this doubt in a measurement, and it is the difference between the measured value and the true value of the quantity being measured.

Note: 'human error' should never be cited as a source of experimental error.

Uncertainties arising from the sensitivity of equipment used are easy to estimate; usually it is half the value of the smallest increment on the instrument scale (basically the number of decimal places to which the equipment can measure). For example, for a two decimal place balance, the smallest increment is 0.01 g, therefore the uncertainty is 0.005 g. When a three decimal place balance is used, the variability of the data reduces, as a three decimal place balance is accurate to within 0.0005 g.

---

**EXAMPLE 3:1**

**Question:** 3.78 g of drug is weighed out on a two decimal and three decimal place balance as shown below. What does this value imply, in terms of the minimum and maximum weight range associated with the measurement on each balance?

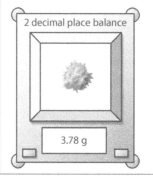

2 decimal place balance

3.78 g

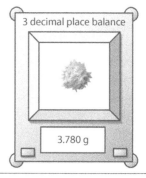

3 decimal place balance

3.780 g

**Answer:**  On a two decimal place balance, the reading is 3.78 g. From the limitation of the balance, the weight of each portion of drug will vary between 3.775 g and 3.785 g. If a three decimal place balance is used, the weight of the drug will be between 3.7795 g and 3.7805 g.

| EXAMPLE 3:2 |
|---|
| **Question:**  What is the volume in this measuring cylinder, including the uncertainty? |

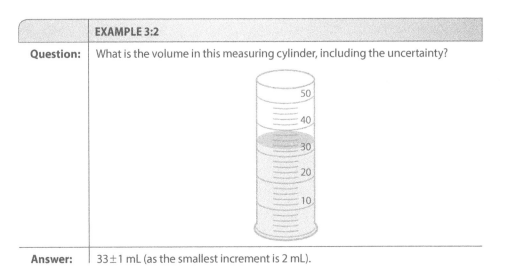

**Answer:**  33±1 mL (as the smallest increment is 2 mL).

## Uncertainty associated with a measurement tool

A useful rule of thumb for estimating the uncertainty associated with a measurement is to determine the smallest increment the device can measure, and then divide this value by two.

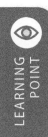

LEARNING POINT

### 3.2.1 Significant figures and reporting data

As we have seen, all measurements are approximations. Therefore, experimental data must be written in a way that reflects the precision with which they are known, and one significant figure should be used to report the uncertainty of a measurement. The significant figures in a number are those digits that have physical meaning. Therefore measurements should be written to the appropriate significant figures, and all definite digits and the first doubtful digit are considered significant. Also leading zeros are not significant figures, whereas trailing zeros are significant figures, as they indicate the precision of the measurement. When writing measurements to an appropriate significant figure, rounding of a measurement may be required; therefore when rounding a measurement, retain as many significant figures as will give only one uncertain figure. When undertaking a calculation, first identify the value in the calculation with the least number of significant figures. Then express the answer to the calculation to the same number of significant figures as the value in the calculation with the least number of significant figures.

| | EXAMPLE 3:3 |
|---|---|
| **Question:** | Round each of the following values to three significant figures: |
| | a) 0.007634. |
| | b) 43.74. |
| | c) 100.66. |
| | d) 0.04455. |
| | e) 22.135±0.001 mg. |
| **Answer:** | a) 0.00763. |
| | b) 43.7. |
| | c) 101. |
| | d) 0.0446. |
| | e) 22.1±0.001 mg. |

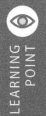

**LEARNING POINT**

### Significant figures

Significant figures are the number of digits in a figure that express the precision of a measurement. General rules with significant figures are:

1.  All non-zero digits are significant.

2.  Any zeros between two significant digits are significant.

3.  For numbers smaller than 1, start counting the number of significant figures from the first non-zero digit.

In calculations, express the answer to a calculation to the same number of significant figures as the value in the calculation with the least number of significant figures.

One significant figure should be used to report the uncertainty of a measurement.

### 3.2.2 Combining uncertainties

Although section 3.2.1 shows how we can estimate an uncertainty associated with a single measurement, often multiple values need to be combined in a measurement or process. Generally, it is better to measure uncertainty directly, through taking repeat measurements and by measuring the standard deviation (see section 3.6.4). However, where this is not possible, uncertainties can be carried through a calculation.

A simple method that can be used is the **range method**. This method adopts the worst case scenario by considering that the measurements to be combined were made on the outer limits of acceptability; the range of the measurement is calculated, and then the uncertainty is half of the calculated range. Therefore this method will give an overestimation of the uncertainty.

| | **EXAMPLE 3:4** |
|---|---|
| **Question:** | $1.6 \pm 0.1$ g of drug is mixed with $5.4 \pm 0.1$ g of diluent and $1.5 \pm 0.1$ g of a binder. What is the total weight and the uncertainty of this blend? |
| **Answer:** | Maximum weight is $(1.6 + 0.1) + (5.4 + 0.1) + (1.5 + 0.1) = 8.8$ g. |
| | Minimum weight is $(1.6 - 0.1) + (5.4 - 0.1) + (1.5 - 0.1) = 8.2$ g. |
| | Total weight $= 1.6 + 5.4 + 1.5 = 8.5$ g. |
| | Range $= 8.8 - 8.2$ g $= 0.6$ g.<br>Therefore the uncertainty $=$ range $\div 2 = \pm 0.3$ g. |

An alternative method to combine uncertainties involves using a technique called **propagation of uncertainty**; this provides a series of functions, the choice of which depends on how the uncertainties are being combined. These are shown in Table 3.1. The uncertainty calculated using this method is smaller than that calculated using the range method, as the range method gives the worst case scenario.

| Action | Calculation of uncertainty |
|---|---|
| **Addition or subtraction**<br><br>$A = B + C$ or $A = B - C$ | Overall error of $A = \sqrt{(error\ B)^2 + (error\ C)^2}$ |
| **Multiplication and division**<br><br>$A = B \times C$ or $A = B \div C$ | Overall error of $A = A \sqrt{(Fractional\ error\ B)^2 + (Fractional\ error\ C)^2}$ |

**Table 3.1** Propagation of uncertainty

| | **EXAMPLE 3:5** |
|---|---|
| **Question:** | Using the propagation of uncertainty method, now calculate the uncertainty associated with Example 3:4. |
| **Answer:** | Uncertainty $= \sqrt{(0.1)^2 + (0.1)^2 + (0.1)^2} = \sqrt{0.03} = 0.17$. |
| | Therefore the uncertainty of the weight is $\pm 0.2$ g (*remember errors are only written to one significant figure*). |

| | **EXAMPLE 3:6** |
|---|---|
| **Question:** | The total weight of a drug and its container is $4.3 \pm 0.1$ g. After removal of the drug, the container had a weight of $0.5 \pm 0.1$ g. What is the weight of the drug that was in the container? |
| **Answer:** | Weight of drug $= 4.3$ g $- 0.5$ g $= 3.8$ g. |
| | Uncertainty $= \sqrt{(0.1)^2 + (0.1)^2} = \sqrt{0.01 + 0.01} = 0.14$. |
| | Therefore the weight of the drug in the container is $3.8 \pm 0.1$ g (*remember errors are only written to one significant figure*). |

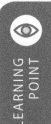

### Reporting physical measurements

With a measurement, an indication of the uncertainty of the measurement must be given. Therefore a physical measurement has two components:

1. A numerical value, which is the best estimate of the quantity measured.

2. The degree of uncertainty associated with this estimated value.

Uncertainties should be written to one significant figure.

The combined uncertainty in a calculation can be estimated using the range method or using the propagation of uncertainty technique.

## 3.3 Accuracy and precision

As already discussed, all measurements have a level of experimental error and uncertainty. When discussing data, **accuracy** refers to the agreement of the measurement with the value expected if there was no error associated (often referred to as the true value). The accuracy of a measurement is defined by how close the measurement is to the true value. An experiment that has very small random and systematic errors will have a high degree of accuracy.

**Precision** refers to the repeatability of a measurement and measures how closely two or more measurements agree with each other. This is sometimes referred to as the 're-peatability' or 'reproducibility' of a measurement. Precision measures random errors. Precision does not measure how close the value is to the true value. As previously described, as random errors produce variations in measurements, experiments with very small random errors have a high degree of precision.

Figure 3.1 gives an example of these terms with regard to tablet weights. The accepted weight for each tablet is 350 mg; if the tablet weight is accurate all the tablets will be close to the accepted weight of 350 mg but not reproducibly 350 mg each time. If the tablets are produced precisely, the tablets will always be the same weight, but not necessarily at the accepted weight of 350 mg. For tablets to be produced at 350 mg, accuracy and precision are required (see Figure 3.1).

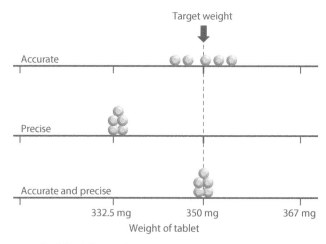

**Figure 3.1** An example of the difference between accuracy and precision.

**EXAMPLE 3:7**

**Question:** Two batches of suspensions have been prepared (Batch A and B; see below); each batch contains five 100 mL bottles containing 200 mg of acyclovir drug in 5 mL. The drug concentration for each suspension is shown in the table below. Which batch (A or B) is more precise and which is more accurate?

| Batch A | Batch B |
| --- | --- |
| 198 mg/5 mL | 193 mg/5 mL |
| 203 mg/5 mL | 192 mg/5 mL |
| 197 mg/5 mL | 191 mg/5 mL |
| 195 mg/5 mL | 193 mg/5 mL |
| 205 mg/5 mL | 192 mg/5 mL |

**Answer:** Batch A shows higher accuracy as the suspensions are close to the accepted concentration of 200 mg/5 mL. Batch B shows higher precision as all the concentrations are similar and reproducible, but this batch is less accurate.

## Accuracy and precision

Accurate measurements are close to the true or accepted value. Accuracy determines how much error is in a method, not how reproducible the method is. Both random and systematic errors affect accuracy.

Precise measurements are closely clustered about a single value, and are repeatable. Highly precise measurements have small variance, but have no relationship to the true value. Random uncertainties contribute to poor precision.

Measurements that are both precise and accurate are repeatable and close to the true or accepted value.

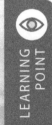

LEARNING POINT

### 3.3.1 Accuracy: absolute error versus relative error

Errors are quantified by associating an uncertainty with a measurement. Whereas precision can be determined by comparing replicate data, accuracy is more difficult, as the true value of a measurement is not usually known; therefore, often the expected value of a measurement is used. The accuracy of a measurement can be quantified mathematically using the **absolute error** and the **relative error**. The **absolute error** is the difference between the observed value and the expected (true) value. This can be expressed as:

Absolute error = observed value − expected value.

| EXAMPLE 3:8 | |
|---|---|
| **Question:** | If a measurement of a drug is 205 mg/5 mL (the observed value) and the expected value is 200 mg/5 mL, what is the absolute error associated with this measurement? |
| **Answer:** | Absolute error = observed value − expected value. |
| | = 205 mg/5 mL − 200 mg/5 mL = 5 mg/5 mL. |

When considering the accuracy of a method or measurement, the measurement with the lowest absolute error can be considered the most accurate. However, the absolute error does not take into account a magnitude of the measurement. Therefore, the **relative error** which is the absolute error divided by the accepted value, can be used to show the error associated with a measurement as a proportion of the expected value:

$$\text{Relative error} = \frac{\text{observed value} - \text{expected value}}{\text{expected value}} = \frac{\text{absolute error}}{\text{expected value}}$$

When calculating the relative error, only the absolute values are used (i.e. the negative signs are ignored). The advantage of using the relative error as opposed to the absolute error is that the accuracies in measurements can be directly compared. This can also be expressed as a percentage value by multiplying the relative value by 100%.

| EXAMPLE 3:9 | |
|---|---|
| **Question:** | From Example 3:8, calculate the relative error and percentage relative error. |
| **Answer:** | $\text{Relative error} = \dfrac{\text{observed value} - \text{expected value}}{\text{expected value}} = \dfrac{\text{absolute error}}{\text{expected value}}$ |
| | $= \dfrac{5\,\text{mg}}{200\,\text{mg}}$ |
| | $= 0.025.$ |
| | % Relative error = 0.025 × 100% = 2.5%. |

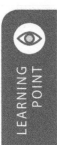

**Absolute error and relative error**

$$\text{Absolute error} = \text{observed value} - \text{expected value}$$

$$\text{Relative error} = \frac{\text{absolute error}}{\text{expected value}}$$

Using the relative error allows the direct comparison of accuracies in measurements.

LEARNING POINT

## 3.4 Data sets: samples and populations

When considering data sets, these can be sample data sets or population data sets. As the terms suggest, a sample tests a part of a population data set, whereas a population data set contains all the data available. A sample of values gives an estimate of a population, which can be useful in large population data sets. For example, when looking around a lecture theatre of pharmacy students, one can determine how many students are within the room and how many students are of a particular gender. This is a population study as all the students within the lecture room have been considered. Alternatively, one could consider only the students sitting in the front two rows of the lecture room, this is a sample study and, although quicker, may not accurately represent the entire population set. Within many studies, it is very difficult or time consuming to undertake population studies; therefore, sample studies are often conducted and this has bearing on some of the methods used to measure variability.

### 3.4.1 Normal distribution

Having collected data as part of a study, and considered the uncertainties associated with the data, it is also important to consider the properties of a data set. In a data set, data can be distributed (spread out) in different ways; it is common for most measurements to cluster around a central value, with no bias. This is described as *normal distribution* or *Gaussian distribution* (after Carl Friedrich Gauss who discovered this probability distribution) with the data giving a 'bell-shaped' curve. Many common attributes such as average height and blood pressure within a population follow normal distributions. Alternatively, it can be skewed or biased to the left or right (see Figure 3.2).

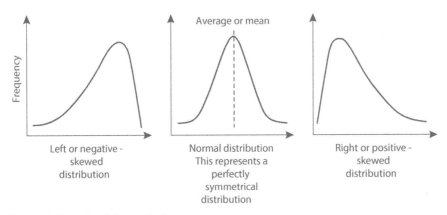

Figure 3.2  Normal and skewed distributions.

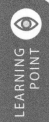

**Normal or Gaussian distribution**

Normally distributed data will be distributed symmetrically about a centre point: 50% of the values will be more than the average of the data set and 50% will be less than the mean.

LEARNING POINT

## 3.5 Calculating the average of data sets

As we have seen, a data set contains a spread of data. Consequently, to work with this data set, the properties of the data set must be summarized. Most commonly this is achieved by considering the central value (or central tendency) of the data and a measure of variability.

### 3.5.1 Mean, median, and mode

As mentioned, most data sets are built of values that are not alike, and the extent to which they are different is an important consideration. To understand and compare data sets, these measurements must be summarized and variability in data measurements must be considered, thereby allowing data sets to be summarized. When considering a data set, its central value may be described using the mean, median, and mode. Each of these represents a single summary value that identifies the central value within a data set, as follows.

- **Mean**—this is often referred to as the average and is the most popular way to describe the central tendency of a data set. It is calculated from the sum of the data values divided by the number of data values, that is you add together all the values in the data set and divide by the number of data points you have. If we have n values in a data set and they have the values $x_1, x_2, x_3 \ldots x_n$, the mean can be calculated as follows:

$$\text{Mean} = \frac{x_1 + x_2 + x_3 + \ldots + x_n}{n}$$

The mean is most appropriate to use when the data are distributed symmetrically around a central point, that is they have a Gaussian distribution.

| EXAMPLE 3:10 | |
|---|---|
| **Question:** | Calculate the mean weight of the tablets from the following sample of eight tablets: |
| | 348 mg, 350 mg, 341 mg, 356 mg, 350 mg, 359 mg, 344 mg, 352 mg. |
| **Answer:** | The **mean** is calculated as follows: |
| | $$\frac{348\text{ mg} + 350\text{ mg} + 341\text{ mg} + 356\text{ mg} + 350\text{ mg} + 359\text{ mg} + 344\text{ mg} + 352\text{ mg}}{8}$$ |
| | Mean = 350 mg. |

- **Median**—this is the data value in the middle of a set of data that has been arranged in order of magnitude. If the data set contains an odd number of data measurements, then the middle measurement in the series is used. If the data set contains an even number of data points, the median is the average of the two middle measurements. When the data set has a Gaussian spread, the mean and median are the same; however, when the data are asymmetrically spread (i.e. do not have a Gaussian distribution), it may be better to use the median rather than the mean, as the median is less affected by outlying data points.

| EXAMPLE 3:11 | |
|---|---|
| **Question:** | From the data set in Example 3:10 calculate the median. |
| **Answer:** | First the data must be arranged in order of magnitude: |
| | 341 mg, 344 mg, 348 mg, 350 mg, 350 mg, 352 mg, 356 mg, 359 mg. |
| | In this data set, the median falls between the fourth and fifth positions, and in this case will be 350 mg. This is the same as the mean as the data are symmetrically distributed. |

- **Mode**—this is the most frequently occurring data measurement occurring within a data set.

If the data set in Example 3:10 is considered, the most frequently occurring data measurement is 350 mg, and therefore in this symmetrically distributed data set, the mean, median, and mode are all equal to 350 mg.

| | EXAMPLE 3:12 |
|---|---|
| **Question:** | Determine the mode from the following set of data: |
| | Concentration in micrograms dm$^{-3}$: 12, 13, 12, 14, 15, 13, 14, 15, 13, 15, 13, 10, 9, 11, 12, 13, and 10. |
| **Answer:** | 13 micrograms dm$^{-3}$. |

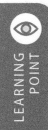

### Mean, median, and mode

**Mean:** This is the average value of a data set. It is calculated from the sum of the data values divided by the number of data values.

**Median:** This is the value in the middle of a set of measurements that has been arranged in order of magnitude.

**Mode:** This is the most frequently occurring data measurement occurring within a set of measurements.

In a data set with normal distribution, the mean, median, and mode are the same.

LEARNING POINT

## 3.6 Measurement of the variability of data

Using the mean, median, and mode, the central tendency of a data set can be described. The next step when summarizing data sets is to show the spread of the data set. The variability of a data set can be measured using a variety of methods.

### 3.6.1 Range

The range is the simplest way to measure variability. The range of a set of measurements is the difference between the largest value and the smallest value in a set of measurements. As the range only considers two measurements from the data set, it is of limited use. In particular, the range of a sample data set may not reflect the variability within a population as it is unlikely that the sample data set will contain the highest and lowest values of the full population data set. To calculate the associated uncertainty, the range is divided by two.

| | EXAMPLE 3:13 |
|---|---|
| **Question:** | To determine the accuracy of a 1.0 cm$^3$ pipette, you measure out 1.0 cm$^3$ of water five times, and weigh the amount of water in each case. The masses of the water are: 0.983 g, 1.022 g, 1.001 g, 0.993 g, and 1.011 g. The density of water is 0.998 cm$^3$ g$^{-1}$. What is the range for these measurements and the associated uncertainty? |

**Answer:** The data range is from 0.983 to 1.022 g.

Therefore the range is $(1.022 - 0.983) = 0.039$.

Therefore the associated uncertainty is $(1.022 - 0.983) \div 2 = 0.039 \div 2 = 0.02$.

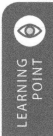

## Range

Range = maximum value – minimum value in a data set.

The associated uncertainty = range ÷ 2.

### 3.6.2 Mean deviation

The amount by which a data point varies from the mean of a data set is known as the deviation. The mean deviation considers how much, on average, each data point within a data set deviates from the mean. However, given that data points can be either higher or lower than the mean value for the data set, this will give positive and negative values for the deviation from the mean. Therefore, as it is the magnitude of the deviation that is important, the algebraic sign of the deviation is ignored (i.e. the negative sign is ignored) and the absolute deviation is used.

Therefore, the mean deviation is calculated as follows:

$$\text{Mean deviation} = \frac{\text{sum of the absolute deviations}}{\text{number of deviations}}$$

| **EXAMPLE 3:14** |
| --- |
| **Question:** What is the mean deviation of the data set in Example 3:13? |
| **Answer:** First you calculate the mean for the data set: |

Mean $= (0.983 + 1.022 + 1.001 + 0.993 + 1.011) \div 5 = 1.002$ g.

Mean deviation $=$

$$\frac{(0.983 - 1.002) + (1.022 - 1.002) + (1.001 - 1.002) + (0.993 - 1.002) + (1.011 - 1.002)}{5}$$

$$= \frac{(0.019) + (0.020) + (0.001) + (0.009) + (0.009)}{5} = 0.0116 \text{ g}.$$

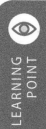

## Mean deviation

This is calculated from the sum of the absolute deviations divided by the number of deviations.

$$\text{Mean deviation} = \frac{\text{sum of the absolute deviations}}{\text{number of deviations}}$$

### 3.6.3 Variance

The variance is described as the mean of the sum of the square of deviations. That is to say, it is obtained by calculating the difference between each value in the data set and the mean (known as the deviation—see section 3.6.2), then squaring the differences, adding them all together, and finally dividing by the number of deviations. Using the square of the deviations eliminates the issue of some deviations being positive and some being negative, as the squares of all real numbers cannot be negative. When considering data sets, these can be sample data sets or population data sets; however, the variances of populations and samples are calculated slightly differently.

The formulae are as follows:

$$\text{Population variance} = \frac{sum\ of\ the\ squares\ of\ the\ deviations}{N} = \frac{\sum (deviations)^2}{N}$$

$$\text{Sample variance} = \frac{sum\ of\ the\ squares\ of\ the\ deviations}{N-1} = \frac{\sum (deviations)^2}{N-1}$$

Where $N=$ the number of values in the data set. As can be seen, when calculating the sample variance, the denominator is $N-1$.

| | |
|---|---|
| **EXAMPLE 3:15** | |
| **Question:** | Calculate the population variance for the data set in Example 3:13. |
| **Answer:** | As in Example 3:14, first you calculate the mean for the data set:<br><br>Mean $=(0.983+1.022+1.001+0.993+1.011)\div5=1.002$ g.<br><br>$$\text{Population variance} = \frac{\sum (deviations)^2}{N}$$<br><br>$$= \frac{(-0.019)^2 + (0.020)^2 + (-0.001)^2 + (-0.009)^2 + (0.009)^2}{5} = 0.000185\ g^2.$$ |

Variance is an important parameter when dealing with experimental uncertainty. It is not a direct measure of the spread of the data as the units are different; the units of variance are the square of the original units of the data value.

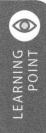

**Variance**

The variance is the mean of the sum of the square of deviations:

$$\text{Population variance} = \frac{sum\ of\ the\ squares\ of\ the\ deviations}{N}$$

$$\text{Sample variance} = \frac{sum\ of\ the\ squares\ of\ the\ deviations}{N-1}$$

LEARNING POINT

### 3.6.4 Standard deviation

Standard deviation (St dev) is the most commonly adopted indicator of the variability of data within a data set. A low standard deviation shows that the data points are close to the mean value, and is therefore a good indication of precision. It does not describe the accuracy of the sample mean. Standard deviation is defined as the square root of the variance; this compensates for the fact that the deviations in the variation were squared. Another advantage of using standard deviation compared with variance is that standard deviation has the same units as the data.

Therefore:

$$\text{Standard deviation} = \sqrt{variance}$$

Given that the deviation of the population and of a sample is calculated using the denominators N and (N–1), respectively, the standard deviation is similarly calculated:

$$\text{Standard deviation of a population} = \sqrt{\frac{\sum (deviation)^2}{N}}$$

$$\text{Standard deviation of a sample} = \sqrt{\frac{\sum (deviation)^2}{N-1}}$$

| EXAMPLE 3:16 | |
|---|---|
| **Question:** | Calculate the standard deviation for the data set in Example 3:13. |
| **Answer:** | Standard deviation $= \sqrt{variance} = \sqrt{0.000185} = 0.0136\,\text{g}$. |

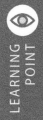

**LEARNING POINT**

**Standard deviation**

**Standard deviation** describes the spread of values in a sample or population. It does not describe the accuracy of the mean. Standard deviation is calculated by taking the square root of the variance.

$$\text{Standard deviation} = \sqrt{variance}$$

Assuming the data are normally distributed, if the mean and the standard deviation of a data set are known, then any value within the data set is:

- Likely to be within 1 standard deviation of the mean value (68 out of 100 should be).
- Very likely to be within 2 standard deviations (95 out of 100 should be).
- Almost certainly within 3 standard deviations (997 out of 1000 should be).

### 3.6.5 Standard error

The standard error of the mean (SEM) is also a commonly used term. This term considers the variability of a set of mean values, calculated from individual groups of measurements that have been taken from a population. Therefore standard error does not describe the variability from individual values.

$$\text{Standard error} = \frac{standard\ deviation}{\sqrt{N}}$$

| EXAMPLE 3:17 | |
|---|---|
| **Question:** | Calculate the standard error for the data set in Example 3:13. |
| **Answer:** | $\text{Standard error} = \dfrac{0.0136}{\sqrt{5}} = 0.00608.$ |

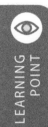

### Standard error of the mean

**Standard error** of the mean (SEM) is the standard deviation of the sample mean. When the sample size increases, SEM decreases.

$$\text{Standard error} = \frac{standard\ deviation}{\sqrt{N}}$$

When reviewing data, check whether the results are reported as **mean±SD** or **mean±SE**. Standard error is often incorrectly used to display data.

**LEARNING POINT**

## 3.6.6 Coefficient of variation

The coefficient of variation (CV) is used to express the degree of variability in a data set in relative terms (e.g. precision of an analytical method). The coefficient of variation expresses the standard deviation as a ratio of the mean:

$$\text{Coefficient of variation }\% = \frac{Standard\ deviation}{mean} \times 100\%.$$

This can be expressed as either a fraction or a percentage.

| EXAMPLE 3:18 | |
|---|---|
| **Question:** | Calculate the % coefficient of variation for the data set in Example 3:13. |
| **Answer:** | $\text{Coefficient of variation }\% = \dfrac{Standard\ deviation}{mean} \times 100\%.$ $= \dfrac{0.0136}{1.002} \times 100\%$ $= 1.36\%.$ |

The coefficient of variation of pharmaceutical analytical methods is normally low; however, for biological samples, for example serum concentrations in patients, it can be high.

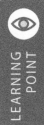

**Coefficient of variation**

The coefficient of variation expresses the standard deviation as a ratio of the mean and can be expressed as either a fraction or a percentage.

$$\text{Coefficient of variation \%} = \frac{Standard\ deviation}{mean} \times 100\%.$$

# 3.7 Self-assessment questions

## 3.7.1 Basic self-assessment questions

This section contains a number of basic self-assessment questions for you to undertake to ensure you have an understanding of the material in this chapter. It is recommended that you undertake all of these calculations **using a calculator** and then check your answers with the answers in section 3.9.

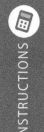

**The use of calculators for the self-assessment questions in this chapter**

It is recommended that you undertake the following calculations using a calculator.

**QUESTION 3.1:**  *A researcher requires 150 mL of water. Rather than using a 200 mL measuring cylinder (which has an associated uncertainty of 0.5 mL), the researcher uses a 50 mL measuring cylinder (which has an associated uncertainty of 0.5 mL) to measure out three lots of 50 mL that are combined to give the researcher a total of 150 mL. Use the range method to estimate the associated uncertainty.*

**QUESTION 3.2:**  *How many significant figures do the following values contain?*

    *a) 0.00528.*

    *b) 0.05028.*

    *c) 0.050280.*

    *d) 5.40.*

    *e) 2008.428.*

    *f) 0.001.*

    *g) 0.1001.*

**QUESTION 3.3:**   *2.6±0.1 g of drug is mixed with 58.5±0.2 g of diluent. What is the total weight and the uncertainty of this blend?*

**QUESTION 3.4:**   *The total weight of ibuprofen and its container is 123±0.3 kg. After removal of the drug, the container had a weight of 0.78±0.1 kg. What is the weight of ibuprofen that was in the container?*

**QUESTION 3.5:**   *In an experiment you weigh out 1.02 g of drug on a two decimal place balance and dissolve this completely in 100±0.5 mL of water. What is the uncertainty associated with the weight of the drug and the resultant drug solution?*

**QUESTION 3.6:**   *A 500 mL infusion bag was prepared to contain 1000 mg vancomycin. Analysis of the contents determined that the infusion bag contained 989 mg vancomycin. What was the absolute error, the relative error, and percentage relative error associated with this measurement?*

**QUESTION 3.7:**   *As part of an experiment you are requested to measure the absorbance of a new drug in solution. You measure the absorbance five times, and the absorbances within the data set are: 0.113, 0.110, 0.117, 0.114, and 0.117. Calculate the mean, median, and mode for this data set.*

**QUESTION 3.8:**   *Using the data set in Question 3.7, calculate the population variance and standard deviation of the data set.*

**QUESTION 3.9:**   *Using the data set in Question 3.7, calculate the SEM and CV% of the data set.*

**QUESTION 3.10:** *Consider the following sample data set:*

  • *Mass (in g) of powder mix: 12.1, 12.2, 12.1, 11.8, and 12.0.*

*Calculate the following:*

  a) *Mean, median, mode.*

  b) *Mean deviation.*

  c) *Variance.*

  d) *Standard deviation.*

  e) *Standard error.*

  f) *% coefficient of variation.*

**QUESTION 3.11:** *Consider the following data set for student exam performance for five students from a student cohort:*

  • *80%, 55%, 70%, 90%, 55%.*

*Calculate the following (assuming this is a sample set):*

  a) *Mean, median, mode.*

  b) *Mean deviation.*

  c) *Variance.*

  d) *Standard deviation.*

  e) *Standard error.*

  f) *% coefficient of variation.*

**QUESTION 3.12:**   *The following serum concentrations of fluoxetine were collected:*

  • *Concentration (ng/mL): 200, 280, 220, 250, 220.*

  *Calculate the following (assume this is a sample data set):*

  a) *Mean, median, mode.*

  b) *Mean deviation.*

  c) *Variance.*

  d) *Standard deviation.*

  e) *Standard error.*

  f) *% coefficient of variation.*

**QUESTION 3.13:**   *An elixir containing 4.00 mg of drug in each 5 mL is tested using three different drug quantification methods. The results are presented in the table below. Calculate the mean and standard deviation for each method. From this, which method gives the most accurate method? Which method has the most precise measurement? (Treat this data as a population data set).*

| Drug quantification method | | |
| --- | --- | --- |
| **HPLC** | **UV Spectroscopy** | **Colorimetric assay** |
| 4.03 mg/mL | 3.81 mg/mL | 5.46 mg/mL |
| 4.01 mg/ml | 3.92 mg/ml | 5.53 mg/mL |
| 3.93 mg/mL | 3.88 mg/mL | 4.91 mg/mL |
| 3.90 mg/mL | 3.77 mg/mL | 6.11 mg/mL |
| 4.05 mg/mL | 3.92 mg/mL | 5.99 mg/mL |

### 3.7.2  Running case studies

**QUESTION 3.14:**

*Since moving into a homeless hostel Marcus has become worried about his weight. He weighs himself every morning for a week and gets the following information. He comes to the pharmacy and asks you to help him calculate his average weight and to explain why his weight is fluctuating daily. Calculate his average weight, the range of these measurements, and the associated standard deviation. Explain to Marcus why his weight varies.*

| Day | Weight |
| --- | --- |
| Monday | 61.0 kg |
| Tuesday | 62.1 kg |
| Wednesday | 61.6 kg |
| Thursday | 62.0 kg |
| Friday | 61.0 kg |
| Saturday | 61.5 kg |
| Sunday | 60.9 kg |

ANSWERS TO SELF-ASSESSMENT QUESTIONS

**QUESTION 3.15:**

*While Marcus is in the pharmacy, you measure his height, which is 1.62 m. The smallest increment on the height meter is 1 cm. What is the uncertainty associated with this measurement?*

## 3.8 Summary

Variability in measurements is unavoidable. It results from a combination of random and systematic uncertainties and errors. Uncertainty is a quantification of this uncertainty in a measurement, and it is the difference between the measured value and the true or expected value of the quantity measured. Therefore, a physical measurement has two components, a numerical value that is the best estimate of the measurement and the degree of uncertainty associated with the measurement. The numerical value of the measurement should be written to the appropriate number of significant figures to express the precision of the measurement. Precision is a measure of the reproducibility of the measurement, whereas accuracy is a measure of how close the measurement is to the accepted value. Accuracy can be quantified by calculating the relative error in a measurement, whereas precision can be quantified by calculating the variation in a set of measurements. To allow the comparison of data sets, the data set should be summarized. This involves calculating the central tendency of the data and the variability. To achieve this there are a selection of methods that can be employed including calculation of the mean deviation, variance, standard deviation, standard error, and coefficient of variation. These methods are referred to as descriptive statistics.

## 3.9 Answers to self-assessment questions

This section contains the worked answers for the self-assessment questions within section 3.7.

**The use of calculators for the self-assessment questions in this chapter**

It is recommended that you undertake the following calculations using a calculator.

INSTRUCTIONS

**QUESTION 3.1:** *A researcher requires 150 mL of water. Rather than using a 200 mL measuring cylinder (which has an associated uncertainty of 0.5 mL), the researcher uses a 50 mL measuring cylinder (which has an associated uncertainty of 0.5 mL) to measure out three lots of 50 mL that are combined to give the researcher a total of 150 mL. Use the range method to estimate the associated uncertainty.*

**ANSWER:** 1.5 mL.

**QUESTION 3.2:** *How many significant figures do the following values contain?*

    *a) 0.00528.*

    *b) 0.05028.*

    *c) 0.050280.*

    *d) 5.40.*

    *e) 2008.428.*

    *f) 0.001.*

    *g) 0.1001.*

**ANSWER:**

    a) 0.00528 (3 significant figures).

    b) 0.05028 (4 significant figures).

    c) 0.050280 (5 significant figures).

    d) 5.40 (3 significant figures).

    e) 2008.428 (7 significant figures).

    f) 0.001 (1 significant figure).

    g) 0.1001 (4 significant figures).

**QUESTION 3.3:** *$2.6 \pm 0.1$ g of drug is mixed with $58.5 \pm 0.2$ g of diluent. What is the total weight and the uncertainty of this blend?*

**ANSWER:** $61.1 \pm 0.2$ g.

**QUESTION 3.4:** *The total weight of ibuprofen and its container is $123 \pm 0.3$ kg. After removal of the drug, the container had a weight of $0.78 \pm 0.1$ kg. What is the weight of ibuprofen that was in the container?*

**ANSWER:** $122.2 \pm 0.3$ kg.

**QUESTION 3.5:** *In an experiment you weigh out 1.02 g of drug on a two decimal place balance and dissolve this completely in $100 \pm 0.5$ mL of water. What is the uncertainty associated with the weight of the drug and the resultant drug solution?*

**ANSWER:** The uncertainty of the drug mass is 0.005 g and therefore the resulting solution has a concentration of $10.2 \pm 0.07$ mg/mL.

**QUESTION 3.6:** *A 500 mL infusion bag was prepared to contain 1000 mg vancomycin. Analysis of the contents determined that the infusion bag contained 989 mg vancomycin. What was the absolute error, the relative error, and percentage relative error associated with this measurement?*

**ANSWER:** The absolute error is 11 mg, the relative error is 0.011, and the percentage relative error is 1.1%.

**QUESTION 3.7:** *As part of an experiment you are requested to measure the absorbance of a new drug in solution. You measure the absorbance five times, and the absorbances within the data set are: 0.113, 0.110, 0.117, 0.114, and 0.117. Calculate the mean, median, and mode for this data set.*

ANSWER: The mean is 0.114, the median is 0.114, and the mode is 0.117.

**QUESTION 3.8:** *Using the data set in Question 3.7, calculate the population variance and standard deviation of the data set.*

ANSWER: The population variance is $6.96 \times 10^{-6}$, and the standard deviation is 0.00264.

**QUESTION 3.9:** *Using the data set in Question 3.7, calculate the SEM and CV% of the data set.*

ANSWER: The SEM is 0.00118 and the CV% is 2.31%.

**QUESTION 3.10:** *Consider the following sample data set:*

- *Mass (in g) of powder mix: 12.1, 12.2, 12.1, 11.8, and 12.0.*

*Calculate the following:*

a) *Mean, median, mode.*

b) *Mean deviation.*

c) *Variance.*

d) *Standard deviation.*

e) *Standard error.*

f) *% coefficient of variation.*

ANSWER:
a) Mean=12.04 g, median=12.1 g, and mode=12.1 g.

b) Mean deviation=0.112 g.

c) Variance=0.0230.

d) Standard deviation=0.152 g.

e) Standard error=0.0678 g.

f) % coefficient of variation=1.26%.

**QUESTION 3.11:** *Consider the following data set for student exam performance for five students from a student cohort:*

- *80%, 55%, 70%, 90%, 55%.*

*Calculate the following (assuming this is a sample set):*

a) *Mean, median, mode.*

b) *Mean deviation.*

c) *Variance.*

d) *Standard deviation.*

e) *Standard error.*

f) *% coefficient of variation.*

**ANSWER:**
a) Mean = 70%, median = 70%, mode = 55%.
b) Mean deviation = 12%.
c) Variance = 238.
d) Standard deviation = 15.4%.
e) Standard error = 6.89%.
f) % coefficient of variation = 22%.

**QUESTION 3.12:** *The following serum concentrations of fluoxetine were collected:*

- Concentration (ng/mL): 200, 280, 220, 250, 220.

*Calculate the following (assume this is a sample data set):*
a) *Mean, median, mode.*
b) *Mean deviation.*
c) *Variance.*
d) *Standard deviation.*
e) *Standard error.*
f) *% coefficient of variation.*

**ANSWER:**
a) Mean = 234 ng/mL, median = 220 ng/mL, mode = 220 ng/mL.
b) Mean deviation = 24.8 ng/mL.
c) Variance = 980.
d) Standard deviation = 31.3 ng/mL.
e) Standard error = 14.0 ng/mL.
f) % coefficient of variation = 13.4%.

**QUESTION 3.13:** *An elixir containing 4.00 mg of drug in each 5 mL is tested using three different drug quantification methods. The results are presented in the table below. Calculate the mean and standard deviation for each method. From this, which method gives the most accurate method? Which method has the most precise measurement? (Treat this data as a population data set).*

| Drug quantification method | | |
| --- | --- | --- |
| HPLC | UV Spectroscopy | Colorimetric assay |
| 4.03 mg/mL | 3.81 mg/mL | 5.46 mg/mL |
| 4.01 mg/mL | 3.92 mg/mL | 5.53 mg/mL |
| 3.93 mg/mL | 3.88 mg/mL | 4.91 mg/mL |
| 3.90 mg/mL | 3.77 mg/mL | 6.11 mg/mL |
| 4.05 mg/mL | 3.92 mg/mL | 5.99 mg/mL |

**ANSWER:**

| Drug quantification method | | |
|---|---|---|
| **HPLC** | **UV Spectroscopy** | **Colorimetric assay** |
| 4.03 mg/mL | 3.81 mg/mL | 5.46 mg/mL |
| 4.01 mg/mL | 3.92 mg/mL | 5.53 mg/mL |
| 3.93 mg/mL | 3.88 mg/mL | 4.91 mg/mL |
| 3.90 mg/mL | 3.77 mg/mL | 6.11 mg/mL |
| 4.05 mg/mL | 3.92 mg/mL | 5.99 mg/mL |
| **Mean** 3.98 mg/mL | 3.86 mg/mL | 5.60 mg/mL |
| **Standard deviation** 0.0585 mg/mL | 0.0603 mg/mL | 0.427 mg/mL |

The HPLC method gives a mean value closest to the expected value and can be considered the most accurate. The standard deviation can be taken as an indicator of precision, and the HPLC assay offers the lowest standard deviation and therefore can also be considered the most precise method.

**QUESTION 3.14:**

*Since moving into a homeless hostel Marcus has become worried about his weight. He weighs himself every morning for a week and gets the following information. He comes to the pharmacy and asks you to help him calculate his average weight and to explain why his weight is fluctuating daily. Calculate his average weight, the range of these measurements, and the associated standard deviation. Explain to Marcus why his weight varies.*

| Day | Weight |
|---|---|
| Monday | 61.0 kg |
| Tuesday | 62.1 kg |
| Wednesday | 61.6 kg |
| Thursday | 62.0 kg |
| Friday | 61.0 kg |
| Saturday | 61.5 kg |
| Sunday | 60.9 kg |

**ANSWER:**

Based on the above data Marcus's average weight is 61.4±0.5 kg; the data range is from 60.9 to 62.1 kg. It is normal for our weight to fluctuate daily (and is dependent on eating, drinking, urinating, and having a bowel movement); this combined with the accuracy/precision of scales used can lead to the variations seen in body weight when measured every day.

**QUESTION 3.15:**

*While Marcus is in the pharmacy, you measure his height, which is 1.62 m. The smallest increment on the height meter is 1 cm. What is the uncertainty associated with this measurement?*

**ANSWER:**

Based on the above data, Marcus's height is 1.62±0.005 m.

# Maths supporting the science of pharmacy

# 4

## 4.1 Chapter introduction

Within this chapter we continue with the examination of calculations relating to the core pharmaceutical sciences by discussing displacement, freezing points, osmolarity, and osmolality. These are all key factors that influence the formulation of medicines and need to be considered in the preparation of a range of products including dry powder antibiotics, injections for reconstitution, suppositories, and pessaries. The clinical impact of isotonicity and serum osmolality is also considered, and ways to prepare isotonic solutions are outlined.

## 4.2 Displacement values and volumes

When a solid is added to a liquid it will add volume, even when dissolved. The amount of solid added, combined with the characteristics of the solid, will dictate how much volume this solid occupies and therefore adds to the total volume. For example, if we dissolve 5 mg of a solid in 50 mL of water, the final volume of the solution will most likely be very close to 50 mL. However, if we were to dissolve 5 g of the solid, an increase in the final volume may be more obvious. Therefore in the formulation and preparation of medicines, we need to consider the impact of adding solids to liquids in terms of final volumes and concentrations, and ensure that medicines are made to the required concentrations.

### 4.2.1 Displacement values of solids in liquids

In practice, many solutions and suspensions are prepared by reconstituting solids with a diluent prior to being given to the patient. For example, drug powders for injection require reconstitution with water for injection, or the reconstitution of dry powders with water to form oral suspensions. When these powders are reconstituted, the final volume of the injection can be greater than the volume of liquid that was added to the powder. This volume difference is known as the **displacement volume**. The displacement volume will depend on the medicine, the brand, and the amount reconstituted. The displacement volume is quoted as the volume displaced by a certain weight or per total container.

The simplest way to accommodate the displacement volume is to consider it as part of the final volume. Therefore the displacement volume is subtracted from the total volume of fluid that would be used to reconstitute the vial. Table 4.1 gives some example displacement volumes for IV antibiotics and volumes to be added. It is important to note that the displacement volumes are brand specific, so different brands of the same antibiotic may have different displacement volumes.

As noted, the displacement volume not only depends on the drug, but also the brand (which will also consider excipients added) has an impact. Therefore oral suspensions, which tend to contain a range of excipients to improve stability and palatability (colourings, flavourings, sweeteners) have larger displacement volumes than injections that contain limited excipients. Indeed for some injections for reconstitution, displacement volume can be negligible.

| Drug | Displacement value | Final volume required | Volume of diluent to be added | Final concentration |
|---|---|---|---|---|
| Amoxicillin (Amoxil®) 500 mg | 0.4 mL | 5 mL | 4.6 mL | 100 mg/mL |
| Ceftazidime (Fortum®) 1 g | 0.9 mL | 10 mL | 9.1 mL | 100 mg/mL |
| Co-Amoxiclav (Augmentin®) 600 mg | 0.5 mL | 10 mL | 9.5 mL | 60 mg/mL |
|  |  | 12 mL | 11.5 mL | 50 mg/mL |
| Flucloxacillin (CP Pharma) 500 mg | 0.4 mL | 10 mL | 9.6 mL | 50 mg/mL |
| Vancomycin (Hospira) 500 mg | 0.32 mL | 10 mL | 9.68 mL | 50 mg/mL |

4 Source: National Policy for the Administration of Intravenous Medication by Registered Nurses and Midwives, 2013.

**Table 4.1** Examples of displacement values for IV antibiotics[4]

| | EXAMPLE 4:1 |
|---|---|
| Question: | The reconstitution instructions for a dry powder of ampicillin to be prepared as oral suspension require the addition of 78 mL of water to give a final volume of 100 mL at a concentration of 125 mg ampicillin in 5 mL. What is the displacement volume for the suspension powder and the total ampicillin content of the suspension product? |
| Answer: | The volume occupied by the powder is the final volume – the volume added.<br><br>Therefore 100 mL – 78 mL = 22 mL/container content.<br><br>The concentration is 125 mg/5 mL, the total volume is 100 mL, therefore the total drug content is 2500 mg. |

| **EXAMPLE 4:2** | |
|---|---|
| **Question:** | A vial containing 3.5 mg of a sterile powder of the monoclonal antibody bortezomib (Velcade) is reconstituted with 3.5 mL of 0.9% sodium chloride for injection. A drug concentration of 1 mg/mL results. What is the displacement volume? |
| **Answer:** | 1 mg/mL is equivalent to 3.5 mg/3.5 mL. Therefore the volume occupied by the bortezomib may be considered negligible. |

| **EXAMPLE 4:3** | |
|---|---|
| **Question:** | Cefuroxime, when reconstituted with 1.8 mL of water for injection, gives a solution of 250 mg in 2 mL. What is the displacement volume for cefuroxime? |
| **Answer:** | The amount of water added was 1.8 mL and the final volume that resulted was 2 mL, therefore the displacement volume is 0.2 mL/250 mg. |

| **EXAMPLE 4:4** | |
|---|---|
| **Question:** | When a vial containing an antibiotic is reconstituted with a volume of 0.9 mL of sterile water for injection, the resulting solution contains 20 mg/mL of drug and the final volume is 1 mL. Calculate the drug content in the vial and its displacement volume. |
| **Answer:** | The total volume is 1 mL and the concentration is 20 mg/mL. Therefore the drug content is 20 mg. 0.9 mL of water was added to the powder to give a total volume of 1 mL, therefore the displacement volume is 0.1 mL/20 mg. |

Examples 4:1 to 4:4 show that the displacement volume can vary widely depending on the formulation. When the complete vial/volume is given to the patient in one dose, the displacement volume need not be accounted for (as the total volume and hence drug content will still be administered). However, often part of the total volume is given, for example for smaller children and neonates. Therefore if the displacement volume is not taken into account, this can result in under dosing.

| **EXAMPLE 4:5** | |
|---|---|
| **Question:** | Using the information in Example 4:3, calculate the dose in 1 mL of the cefuroxime if 2 mL of water for injection was added. |
| **Answer:** | The total volume would be 2 mL + the displacement value of 0.2 mL, giving a total volume of 2.2 mL. |
| | The concentration would be 250 mg in 2.2 mL, equivalent to a dose of 114 mg in 1 mL, rather than 125 mg in 1 mL. |

A table of displacement values is also published in *The Pharmaceutical Codex*. In some cases the displacement value of a drug is given for a specific quantity of drug. In these cases, the displacement volume for the appropriate amount of drug should be calculated.

| | **EXAMPLE 4:6** |
|---|---|
| **Question:** | Diamorphine has a displacement value of 0.06 mL/5 mg. You are required to prepare 40 mL of a solution at a concentration of 20 mg/mL. What volume of diluent should you add to give you a volume of 40 mL at the required concentration? |
| **Answer:** | First, calculate the total weight of drug required: 20 mg × 40 mL = 800 mg. |
| | 800 mg of drug will displace 9.6 mL. |
| | Therefore 30.4 mL of diluent should be added to 800 mg of diamorphine to give 40 mL of solution at 20 mg/mL. |

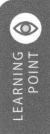

### Displacement volume

The addition of a solid to a liquid adds to the final volume. The volume it adds is known as the displacement volume. The displacement volume will depend on the type and amount of drug and excipients present.

LEARNING POINT

### 4.2.2 Displacement values of solids incorporated into other solids

A range of dosage forms require the incorporation of one solid into another, for example the preparation of suppositories and pessaries. In general these are prepared from a solid base, where the drug is added.

In the extemporaneous preparation of suppositories, the moulds are a fixed shape and volume and are calibrated on the amount of base they contain. This is normally theobroma oil, although other moulds are available. Therefore, a 2 g nominal mould will have a volume appropriate to hold 2 g of theobroma oil. This will have implications when other ingredients are added to the mixtures, as solids with different densities will occupy different volumes within the moulds. When these solids are mixed, the drug will occupy space and the space it adds will depend on its density.

- If the drug and the solid base have the same density, it will displace the equivalent weight of the base.
- If the density of the drug is greater than the base, it will displace a proportionally smaller weight of base.
- If the density of the drug is less than the base, it will displace proportionally more base.

The amount of drug that would displace 1 g of the suppository base is known as the **displacement value**. Therefore, when calculating the amount of base to prepare suppositories or pessaries, the amount of base displaced must be calculated and it will depend on the density of the drug being added and the base used in the formulation. *The Pharmaceutical Codex* contains a list of drugs and their displacement value for 1 g of theobroma oil, which is the traditional suppository base and some examples are given in Table 4.2. Thus, 1.1 g of aspirin will displace 1 g of theobroma oil; similarly 4.7 g of zinc oxide (which has a relatively high density) will displace 1 g of base.

| Drug | Displacement value |
|---|---|
| Aspirin BP | 1.1 |
| Codeine phosphate BP | 1.1 |
| Hydrocortisone BP | 1.5 |
| Morphine hydrochloride BP | 1.6 |
| Paracetamol BP | 1.5 |
| Phenobarbital sodium BP | 1.2 |
| Zinc oxide BP | 4.7 |

5 Source: *The Pharmaceutical Codex* 12th Ed, 1994.

**Table 4.2** Examples of displacement values for theobroma oil[5]

|  | **EXAMPLE 4:7** |
|---|---|
| **Question:** | Aspirin has a displacement value in theobroma oil of 1.1. If the suppository is to contain 0.4 g of aspirin, what weight of theobroma oil will be needed to prepare a suppository using a 2 g nominal mould? |
| **Answer:** | 1.1 g of aspirin displaces 1 g of theobroma oil. |
|  | Therefore 0.4 g will displace $0.4 \div 1.1 = 0.36$ g of theobroma oil. |
|  | Therefore weight of theobroma oil needed $= 2$ g $- 0.36$ g $= 1.64$ g. |

Note the total weight of the suppository is 2.04 g, which is greater than the nominal weight of a suppository, that is 2 g. This is because the displacement value of aspirin is greater than 1.

|  | **EXAMPLE 4:8** |
|---|---|
| **Question:** | You are asked to prepare six suppositories using 2 g nominal moulds, each containing 100 mg of paracetamol and using theobroma oil as the base. The displacement value of paracetamol is 1.5. To allow for wastage, you calculate for eight suppositories. What is the mass of paracetamol and base you require? |
| **Answer:** | Mass of paracetamol $= 8 \times 100$ mg $= 800$ mg. |
|  | The displacement value of paracetamol is 1.5. |
|  | Therefore, 1.5 g of paracetamol displaces 1 g of base. |
|  | Therefore, 0.8 g of paracetamol will displace 0.53 g of base. |
|  | Total amount of base $= (8 \times 2g) - 0.53$ g $= 15.47$ g. |

| | **EXAMPLE 4:9** |
|---|---|
| **Question:** | A prescription requires 40 mg of phenobarbital sodium suppositories prepared using 2 g nominal moulds. What would be the displacement value if it is known that six suppositories with the required drug added weigh 12.04 g? |
| **Answer:** | Six suppositories without drug = 12.00 g. |
| | Six suppositories with drug = 12.04 g. |
| | Amount of drug in the suppositories = $0.04 \times 6 = 0.24$ g. |
| | Therefore, amount of base in the suppositories = $12.04 - 0.24 = 11.8$ g. |
| | Therefore, the amount of base displaced by the drug = $12 - 11.8$ g = 0.2 g. |
| | Therefore, 0.2 g of base was displaced by 0.24 g of drug. |
| | Therefore, 1 g of base will be displaced by 1.2 g of drug. |
| | Therefore, the displacement value is 1.2. |

In the above examples the base used was theobroma oil and the displacement values given were determined for theobroma oil; the displacement value is dependent on the density of the base used. Therefore, if other bases are used the displacement value for a given drug may be different. Many synthetic bases have the same density as theobroma oil so the same displacement values can be used in calculations. For example, the displacement value of Witepsol H15 is taken to be the same as theobroma oil. However, glycol gelatin base is denser than theobroma oil and 1.2 g of glycol gelatin base has a volume equivalent to 1 g of theobroma oil. Given that nominal suppository moulds are based on theobroma oil, a nominal 1 g mould will hold 1 g of theobroma oil or 1.2 g of glycol gelatin base. Similarly, a 2 g nominal mould will hold 2 g of theobroma oil or 2.4 g of glycol gelatin base.

| | **EXAMPLE 4:10** |
|---|---|
| **Question:** | Aspirin has a displacement value in theobroma oil of 1.1. If the suppository is to contain 0.4 g of aspirin, calculate what weight of drug and glycol gelatin will be needed to prepare six suppositories using a nominal 2 g mould. Assume that a nominal 1 g mould will hold 1.2 g of glycol gelatin base. |
| **Answer:** | Amount of drug required is $6 \times 0.4$ g = 2.4 g. |
| | Amount of theobroma base displaced = $2.4 \div 1.1 = 2.18$ g. |
| | Total amount of theobroma base = $(6 \times 2 \text{ g}) - 2.18$ g = 9.82 g. |
| | However, the displacement value is for theobroma oil not glycol gelatin. |
| | Given that 1.2 g of glycol gelatin is equivalent to 1 g of theobroma base, the amount of glycol gelatin base is: |
| | $1.2((6 \times 2 \text{ g}) - 2.18 \text{ g}) = 11.78$ g of glycol gelatin is required. |

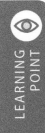

LEARNING POINT

**Displacement value**

This is the number of parts by weight of a drug which displaces one part by weight of the base (theobroma oil BP).

A nominal mould size refers to the weight of theobroma oil which fills the mould. Many synthetic bases have the same density as theobroma oil so the same displacement values can be used in calculations.

If the amount of drug to be incorporated into the base is given as a percentage, the displacement value does not need to be considered.

## 4.3 Iso-osmotic and isotonic solutions: considerations for formulations

Osmotic pressure is caused by a difference in concentration of solutes across a semiper-meable membrane. As the solute cannot cross the membrane via diffusion, the solvent crosses the membrane via osmosis. This movement of solvent results in osmotic pres-sure. A solution is iso-osmotic if the concentration of solute on both sides of the semi-permeable membrane is the same and there is no net movement of water (Figure 4.1A). A hypo-osmotic solution has a lower solute concentration and therefore there is a net movement of solvent from this solution across the semipermeable membrane (Figure 4.1B). A hyper-osmotic solution has a higher concentration of solute, thus there is a net movement of water to this solution (Figure 4.1C).

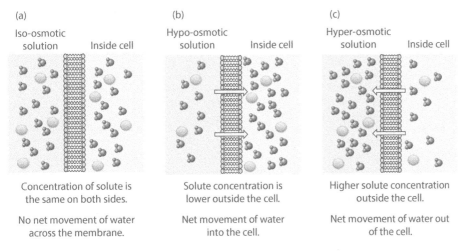

(a)

Iso-osmotic solution          Inside cell

Concentration of solute is the same on both sides.

No net movement of water across the membrane.

(b)

Hypo-osmotic solution          Inside cell

Solute concentration is lower outside the cell.

Net movement of water into the cell.

(c)

Hyper-osmotic solution          Inside cell

Higher solute concentration outside the cell.

Net movement of water out of the cell.

**Figure 4.1** Iso-osmotic and isotonic solutions.

With physiological solutions, isotonicity is often considered. For example, ophthalmic, nasal, and parenteral solutions should be *isotonic*. That is to say these solutions should have the same osmotic pressure as the body fluid with which they are mixed. This will mean there is no net movement of solvent across the semipermeable membrane of cells. If a solution is *hypertonic*, the solution will have a higher osmotic pressure than that of body fluids and when injected intravenously this will cause water to flow out of red blood cells, causing cells to shrink (crenulation). If a solution is *hypotonic*, the solution outside the red blood cells will be less concentrated than inside the cells. Because of this, water flows into the cells. This in turn can cause cells to burst (lysis) (Table 4.3). Therefore, isotonicity is an important factor in the formulation of solutions to avoid irritation or damage at the site of administration.

Body fluids, including blood and lacrimal fluid, normally have an osmotic pressure that is described as corresponding to a 0.9% w/v solution of sodium chloride. The body also attempts to keep the osmotic pressure of the contents of the gastrointestinal (GI) tract at about this level, but there the normal range is much wider than that of most body fluids. The osmotic pressure of a drug solution will depend mainly on the concentration of electrolytes and non-electrolytes in the solution. For example, 0.9% sodium chloride has the same osmotic pressure as blood and tears, and therefore 0.9% w/v NaCl is isotonic with blood. There can be situations where non-isotonic solutions can be used therapeutically; for example, hypotonic solutions such as 0.45% NaCl can be used to aid urine output. Hypertonic solutions (e.g. 5% dextrose in normal saline solution) may be given to patients with hyponatremia and oedema.

| Solution | Description | Effect on cell |
| --- | --- | --- |
| Isotonic | The solution outside the cell is the same osmotic pressure as inside the cell, therefore there is no net gain or loss of water by the cell. | No effect |
| Hypertonic | The solution outside the cell has a higher osmotic pressure than inside the cell. Water moves out of the cell and the cell shrinks. | Crenulation |
| Hypotonic | The solution outside the cell has a lower osmotic pressure than inside the cell. Water moves into the cell causing it to burst. | Cell lysis |

**Table 4.3** The effect of tonicity on red blood cells

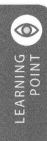

## Isotonic solutions

The tonicity of a solution can be considered as the ability of the solution to cause water movement from one compartment to another.

An isotonic solution is a solution that has the same osmotic pressure as a body fluid. If the osmotic pressure is lower than body fluid, the solution is hypotonic. These solutions can cause cell lysis. Hypertonic solutions have a higher osmotic pressure than a body fluid and can cause shrinkage of red blood cells.

# 4.4 Preparing isotonic solutions

As mentioned, for many routes of administration it is important that the solution is isotonic. Often sodium chloride is used to make a solution isotonic. However other isotonic solutions such as 5% glucose in water and Lactated Ringer's solution (which contains sodium, potassium, calcium, chlorine, and lactate) are also used. Although the tonicity of blood and tears is known, the osmotic pressure of a solution is not easy to measure directly. Therefore in preparing isotonic solutions, methods that consider **freezing point depression, molecular concentration,** or **sodium chloride equivalents** can be used.

## 4.4.1 Freezing point depression

While pure water freezes at 0°C, the presence of salts in water influences the osmolarity and the freezing point of water, and this effect is concentration-dependent. Therefore, the freezing point of a solution can be used to measure its osmolarity. The freezing point of blood serum plasma and tears is –0.52°C. Therefore, an aqueous solution that freezes at –0.52°C is isotonic.

| | EXAMPLE 4:11 |
|---|---|
| **Question:** | 1% w/v of NaCl solution freezes at –0.576°C. What concentration of NaCl (as w/v) is required to prepare an isotonic saline solution with a freezing point of –0.52°C? |
| **Answer:** | –0.576°C is the freezing point of 1% solution.<br>Therefore, $-0.52 \div -0.576 = 0.9\%$ w/v. |

From the above example, we can see that a 0.9% w/v NaCl solution would give an isotonic solution. Using this same principle, the concentration of NaCl required to adjust a hypotonic drug solution to be isotonic can be calculated.

| | EXAMPLE 4:12 |
|---|---|
| **Question:** | 1% w/v of atropine sulfate solution freezes at –0.07°C. What concentration of NaCl (as w/v) is required to make this solution isotonic with blood? Note a 1% w/v of NaCl solution freezes at –0.576°C. |

| **Answer:** | An isotonic solution freezes at −0.52°C. |
|---|---|
| | 1% w/v of atropine sulfate solution freezes at −0.07°C. |
| | The freezing point needs to be reduced by 0.45°C. |
| | −0.576°C is the freezing point of 1% NaCl solution. |
| | Therefore, −0.45 ÷ −0.576 = 0.78% w/v of NaCl is required. |

The above question can also be calculated using the following equation:

$$W = \frac{(0.52 - a)}{b}$$

Where W is the % w/v of adjusting substance in the final solution, *a* is the freezing point depression resulting from the % w/v unadjusted solution, and *b* is the freezing point depression of water caused by 1% w/v of adjusting substance, which in Example 4:12 is NaCl. Therefore, using this equation Example 4:12 is calculated as follows:

Answer: $W = \dfrac{(0.52 - a)}{b}$

$$= \frac{(0.52 - 0.07)}{0.576} = 0.78\% \text{ NaCl is required.}$$

Both methods use the same process and give you the percentage of sodium chloride required; however, the mass of NaCl required will depend on the volume. In some instances the solution required to be isotonic may not be a 1% solution. Therefore, in calculating the freezing point depression, the concentration of the drug solution must be factored in.

| | **EXAMPLE 4:13** |
|---|---|
| **Question:** | 1% w/v of pilocarpine nitrate solution freezes at −0.14°C. What concentration of NaCl (as w/v) is required to make this solution isotonic with blood? What mass of NaCl will be required to prepare a 20 mL solution? Note a 1% w/v of NaCl solution freezes at −0.576°C. |
| **Answer:** | An isotonic solution freezes at −0.52°C. |
| | 1% w/v of pilocarpine nitrate solution freezes at −0.14°C. |
| | The freezing point needs to be reduced by 0.38°C. |
| | Therefore, −0.38 ÷ −0.576 = 0.66% w/v of NaCl is required. |
| | 0.66% w/v NaCl = 0.66 g per 100 mL. |
| | Therefore, for 20 mL = 0.13 g of NaCl is required. |

| | **EXAMPLE 4:14** |
|---|---|
| **Question:** | Calculate how much NaCl is required to make a 10 mL bottle of 1% chloramphenicol eye drops isotonic, given that 1% w/v of chloramphenicol solution freezes at −0.06°C and a 1% w/v of NaCl solution freezes at −0.576°C. |

| | |
|---|---|
| **Answer:** | An isotonic solution freezes at −0.52°C. |
| | 1% w/v of chloramphenicol solution freezes at −0.06°C. |
| | The freezing point needs to be reduced by 0.46°C. |
| | Therefore −0.46 ÷ −0.576 = 0.80% w/v of NaCl is required. |
| | 0.80% w/v NaCl = 0.80 g per 100 mL. |
| | Therefore for 10 mL = 0.08 g of NaCl is required. |

| | |
|---|---|
| **EXAMPLE 4:15** | |
| **Question:** | Calculate the mass of NaCl required to make a 0.5 mL unit dose of pilocarpine 2% eye drops isotonic. Note 1% w/v of pilocarpine solution freezes at −0.14°C and a 1% w/v of NaCl solution freezes at −0.576°C. |
| **Answer:** | An isotonic solution freezes at −0.52°C. |
| | 1% w/v of pilocarpine solution freezes at −0.14°C. |
| | 2% w/v will freeze at −0.14°C × 2 = −0.28°C. |
| | The freezing point needs to be reduced by 0.24°C. |
| | Therefore, −0.24 ÷ −0.576 = 0.42% w/v of NaCl is required. |
| | 0.42% = 0.42 g in 100 mL, therefore for 0.5 mL = 0.0021 g or 2.1 mg NaCl is required. |

## Preparing isotonic solutions—freezing point depression

The presence of salts in water influences the freezing point of water, and this effect is concentration-dependent. The freezing point of blood serum plasma and tears is −0.52°C. Therefore, an aqueous solution that freezes at −0.52°C is isotonic.

The amount of an adjusting substance required to make a solution isotonic can be calculated using proportionality sets or as follows:

$$W = \frac{(0.52 - a)}{b}$$

Where W is the % w/v of adjusting substance in the final solution, $a$ is the freezing point depression of unadjusted solution, and $b$ is the freezing point depression of water caused by 1% w/v of adjusting substance. Often NaCl is used to adjust the tonicity of a solution.

LEARNING POINT

### 4.4.2 Osmolarity and osmolality

Solutions can also be made isotonic with blood by matching the osmolarity of a solution with that of blood. The osmolarity of a solution is based on the total number of osmotically active substances in the solution. The normal range of osmolarity of blood is approximately 275 to 300 mmol/L, that is there are 0.3 moles of osmotically active substances per litre of blood. The SI units used for osmolarity are in mmol/L; however, milliosmole (mOsmol) is also used as the unit to measure osmotic concentration. There are two types of osmotically active substances:

1. Substances that do not dissociate and maintain their molecular structure when they dissolve (i.e. they maintain their molecular structure when dissolved). An example of this is glucose. A 0.3 molar solution of glucose has an osmolarity of 300 mmol/L.

2. Substances that dissociate when they dissolve. For example, a 0.3 molar NaCl solution when fully dissociated forms 0.3 moles of $Na^+$ and 0.3 moles of $Cl^-$. This gives a total of 0.6 moles of active substances in solution, and therefore the solution has an osmolarity of 0.6 mmol/L.

Therefore by knowing the number of osmotically active species in a solution, the osmolarity can be estimated. By matching the osmolarity of the solution to that of blood, solutions will be isotonic and appropriate for injection.

| EXAMPLE 4:16 | |
|---|---|
| **Question:** | What is the osmolarity of 0.9% NaCl? The molecular weight of NaCl is 58.5. |
| **Answer:** | 0.9% NaCl contains 0.9 g in 100 mL, therefore 9 g in 1000 mL. |
| | The number of moles of NaCl in 1 L = weight ÷ molecular weight |
| | = 9 ÷ 58.5 = 0.154 moles. |
| | NaCl has two osmotically active species: $Na^+$ and $Cl^-$, therefore the osmolarity of the solution is 0.308 mol/L or 308 mmol/L. |
| | Note, we have already observed that a 0.9% NaCl solution is isotonic. |

| EXAMPLE 4:17 | |
|---|---|
| **Question:** | What molarity of KCl is isotonic with blood? |
| **Answer:** | The osmolarity of blood = 0.3 mol/L. |
| | KCl has two osmotically active species: $K^+$ and $Cl^-$, therefore a 0.15 molar solution of KCl will be isotonic with blood assuming complete dissociation of KCl. |

| EXAMPLE 4:18 | |
|---|---|
| **Question:** | What is the osmolarity of 0.5% glucose? The molecular weight of glucose is 180 g/mol. |
| **Answer:** | 0.5% glucose contains 0.5 g in 100 mL, therefore 5 g in 1000 mL. |
| | The number of moles of glucose in 1 L = 5 ÷ 180 = 0.028 moles. |
| | Glucose does not dissociate and therefore has one osmotically active species; therefore the osmolarity of the solution is 0.028 mol/L. |

### 4.4.3 Osmolality and clinical relevance

In addition to osmolarity, **osmolality** is a measure of the osmolar concentration per kilogram of solvent and therefore the IS unit is mmol/kg (but mOsmol/kg is still widely used). Clinically, osmolality is commonly used when considering hydration, hyper/hyponatremia, and renal function. Normal serum osmolality is usually taken as 280–295 mOsm/kg. Similarly, urine osmolality is used to evaluate renal function. In the case of decreased renal function, patients may not be able to concentrate urine, resulting in low urine osmolality. An average urine osmolality is around 500-800 mmol/kg. Table 4.4 gives some examples where osmolality can be measured as a clinical indicator.

|  | Serum | Urine |
|---|---|---|
| **Increased osmolality** | Dehydration | Dehydration |
|  | Hyperglycaemia | Inappropriate ADH secretion |
|  | Diabetes insipidus | Hypernatremia |
|  | Uraemia | High protein diet |
|  | Hypernatremia |  |
|  | Ethanol, methanol, or ethylene glycol ingestion |  |
| **Decreased osmolality** | Excess hydration | Diabetes insipidus |
|  | Hyponatremia | Excess fluid intake |
|  | Inappropriate ADH secretion | Acute renal insufficiency |

**Table 4.4** Examples of conditions associated with altered osmolality

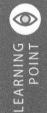

### Osmolarity and osmolality

**Osmolarity** is an expression of osmolar concentration and is defined as the number of osmoles (osmotically active substances) per litre of solution, and it is expressed as mmol/L.

**Osmolality** is a measure of osmolar concentration per kilogram of solvent and is measured in mmol/kg.

A 1 molar solution of glucose has an osmolarity of 1 mol/L as glucose does not dissociate. However, a 1 molar solution of NaCl if fully dissociated has an osmolarity of 2 mol/L, as 1 mole of NaCl dissociates fully in water to give 1 mole of $Na^+$ and 1 mole of $Cl^-$ ions, therefore a total of 2 osmoles in solution.

LEARNING POINT

### 4.4.4 Sodium chloride equivalent method

Sodium chloride is commonly used to adjust the tonicity of solutions and, using this method, sodium chloride equivalents show the concentration of NaCl that would have the same effect on tonicity as 1% of an alternative agent. Examples of sodium chloride equivalents for a range of compounds are provided in Table 4.5. Using this information, any hypotonic solution can be made isotonic by adding the appropriate quantity of sodium chloride.

| Substance | Sodium chloride equivalents |
|---|---|
| Ammonium chloride | 1.08 |
| Atropine sulfate | 0.13 |
| Chlorobutanol | 0.18 |
| Ephedrine hydrochloride | 0.30 |
| Neomycin sulfate | 0.11 |
| Pilocarpine nitrate | 0.22 |
| Zinc chloride | 0.62 |

**Table 4.5** Examples of sodium chloride equivalents

| | **EXAMPLE 4:19** |
|---|---|
| **Question:** | How much sodium chloride is required to make a 1% w/v solution of atropine sulfate solution isotonic? |
| **Answer:** | The sodium chloride equivalent of atropine sulfate is 0.13, that is a 1% solution of atropine sulfate has the same osmotic pressure as a 0.13% solution of sodium chloride. |
| | A 0.9% NaCl solution is considered isotonic, therefore 0.77 g of sodium chloride per 100 mL of a 1% solution of atropine sulfate is required to make the solution isotonic. |

| | **EXAMPLE 4:20** |
|---|---|
| **Question:** | What mass of NaCl should be added to 50 mL of a 1% w/v procaine hydrochloride solution to make it isotonic with blood (sodium chloride equivalent of procaine HCl is 0.21)? |
| **Answer:** | 1% procaine HCl is equivalent to 0.21% NaCl. |
| | 0.9% NaCl is isotonic with blood; therefore 0.69% w/v NaCl is required. |
| | For 100 mL this is 0.69 g, therefore for 50 mL 0.345 g NaCl is required. |

However, this method is not only restricted to the addition of NaCl to prepare an isotonic solution; but also can be used for other compounds.

| | **EXAMPLE 4:21** |
|---|---|
| **Question:** | What mass of dextrose is required to make 100 mL of a 1% w/v ephedrine sulfate solution isotonic with blood? (NaCl equivalent of ephedrine sulfate is 0.23, sodium chloride equivalent of dextrose is 0.16.) |
| **Answer:** | 1% ephedrine sulfate is equivalent to 0.23% NaCl. |
| | 0.9% NaCl is isotonic with blood; therefore 0.67% w/v NaCl is required. |
| | However, dextrose is to be used. 1% dextrose is equivalent to 0.16% NaCl. |
| | Therefore, $0.67 \div 0.16 = 4.2\%$ w/v of dextrose is required. |
| | Thus the mass required for 100 mL is 4.2 g. |

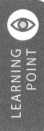

**Sodium chloride equivalent method for adjusting isotonicity**

The sodium chloride equivalent of a substance can be taken as the amount (in % w/v) of sodium chloride that is osmotically equivalent to 1% of the substance.

LEARNING POINT

# 4.5 Self-assessment questions

## 4.5.1 Basic self-assessment questions

This section contains a number of basic self-assessment questions for you to undertake to ensure you have an understanding of the material in this chapter. It is recommended that you undertake all of these calculations **using a calculator** and then check your answers with the answers in section 4.7.

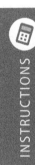

**The use of calculators for the self-assessment questions in this chapter**

It is recommended that you undertake the following calculations using a calculator.

INSTRUCTIONS

**QUESTION 4.1:**   *You add 5 mL of diluent to an ampoule containing 500 mg of amoxicillin. The final volume is 5.4 mL. What is the displacement value for the powder in the ampoule?*

**QUESTION 4.2:**   *The displacement value for diamorphine as a powder for reconstitution is 0.6 mL/5 mg. What volume would 40 mg of diamorphine displace?*

**QUESTION 4.3:**   *You are required to reconstitute a 1 g vial of ceftazidime to a concentration of 100 mg/mL. The powder has a displacement value of 0.9 mL. What volume of water for injection should you add to give you a final volume of 10 mL and a concentration of 100 mg/mL?*

**QUESTION 4.4:**   *You are asked to prepare an IV injection of benzylpenicillin at 150 mg/mL. You have 600 mg vials of benzylpenicillin and the displacement value for this powder is 0.4 mL. What volume of water for injection should you add to the ampoule to achieve the required concentration?*

**QUESTION 4.5:**   *A patient requires an IV injection of meropenem at a concentration of 50 mg/mL. You have 1 g ampoules of meropenem with a displacement value of 0.9 mL. What volume of water for injection should be added to achieve the required concentration?*

**QUESTION 4.6:** *A pharmacist receives a prescription requesting a concentration of an antibiotic suspension to be prepared to a concentration of amoxicillin 200 mg/5 mL. The label for amoxicillin powder for oral suspensions states 68 mL of water should be added to the container to give a final volume of 100 mL, with a concentration of 250 mg amoxicillin per 5 mL of suspension. What volume (in mL) should the pharmacist add to the amoxicillin powder to produce a concentration of 200 mg/5 mL?*

**QUESTION 4.7:** *You are required to prepare six promethazine hydrochloride suppositories each containing 20 mg of drug and using theobroma base and 2 g nominal moulds. You prepare eight suppositories to accommodate wastage. How much drug and base do you require? The displacement value of promethazine hydrochloride is 2.5.*

**QUESTION 4.8:** *You are required to prepare six paracetamol suppositories each containing 500 mg of drug and using theobroma base and 2 g nominal moulds. You prepare eight suppositories to accommodate wastage. How much drug and base do you require? The displacement value of paracetamol is 1.5.*

**QUESTION 4.9:** *In the above preparation you change the base from theobroma oil to glycol gelatin. Assuming that a nominal 1 g mould will hold 1.2 g of glycol gelatin base, how much glycol gelatin base should be used and what will be the weight of each suppository?*

**QUESTION 4.10:** *A prescription requires 150 mg of miconazole nitrate pessaries prepared using a 2 g nominal mould. What would be the displacement value if it is known that six pessaries with the required miconazole nitrate added weigh 12.34 g?*

**QUESTION 4.11:** *1% w/v of chloramphenicol solution freezes at −0.06°C. What concentration of NaCl (as w/v) is required to make this solution isotonic? Note a 1% w/v of NaCl solution freezes at −0.576°C.*

**QUESTION 4.12:** *1% w/v of morphine sulfate solution freezes at −0.08°C and a 1% w/v of NaCl solution freezes at −0.576°C. What concentration of NaCl (as w/v) is required to make this solution isotonic? What mass of NaCl will be required to prepare a 30 mL solution?*

**QUESTION 4.13:** *1% w/v of glucose solution freezes at −0.091°C. What concentration of glucose (as w/v) is required to prepare an isotonic solution with a freezing point of −0.52°C?*

**QUESTION 4.14:** *Calculate how much NaCl is required to make a 10 mL bottle of 0.5% chloramphenicol eye drops isotonic given that 1% w/v of chloramphenicol solution freezes at −0.06°C and a 1% w/v of NaCl solution freezes at −0.576°C.*

**QUESTION 4.15:** *Ephedrine sulfate injection is a sterile solution of ephedrine sulfate in water. Each mL contains 30 mg of ephedrine sulfate. How much sodium chloride is required to make this 1 mL solution isotonic given that 1% w/v of ephedrine sulfate freezes at −0.13°C and a 1% w/v of NaCl solution freezes at −0.576°C?*

**QUESTION 4.16:** *What mass of dextrose is required to produce 200 mL of a solution that is isotonic with blood? The MW of dextrose is 180.*

**QUESTION 4.17:** *What mass of KCl is required to produce 100 mL of a solution that is isotonic with blood? The MW of KCl = 74.5.*

**QUESTION 4.18:** *What molar concentration of NaCl is required to make a 1.5% w/v dextrose solution isotonic with blood? (MW of dextrose is 180.)*

**QUESTION 4.19:** *How much sodium chloride is required to make a 1% w/v solution of a pilocarpine nitrate solution isotonic? (Sodium chloride equivalent of pilocarpine nitrate is 0.22.)*

**QUESTION 4.20:** *What mass of NaCl should be added to 80 mL of a 0.5% w/v ammonium chloride solution to make it isotonic with blood? (Sodium chloride equivalent of ammonium chloride is 1.08.)*

### 4.5.2 Running case studies

**QUESTION 4.21:**

*Marcus has been prescribed 0.5% chloramphenicol eye drugs for a bacterial eye infection. Calculate how much NaCl is required to make a 5 mL isotonic solution given that 1% w/v of chloramphenicol solution freezes at −0.06°C and a 1% w/v of NaCl solution freezes at −0.576°C.*

**QUESTION 4.22:**

*Emma has been given a prescription for an oral antibiotic suspension. The label for powder for oral suspensions states 74 mL of water should be added to the container to give a final volume of 100 mL, at a concentration of 125 mg antibiotic in 5 mL. What is the displacement volume for the suspension powder and the total antibiotic content of the suspension product?*

# 4.6 Summary

It is vital that medicines are prepared to the required concentration. Therefore, when reconstituting solids with a diluent the displacement volume must be considered. The displacement volume depends on the medicine, the brand, and the amount reconstituted, and it is quoted as the volume displaced by a certain weight or per total container. Similarly, a range of dosage forms require the incorporation of one solid into another, for example in the preparation of suppositories and pessaries. The amount of drug that would displace 1 g of the suppository base is known as the displacement value, and this must be taken into account when calculating the amount of base to prepare suppositories or pessaries.

The presence of dissolved substances in a solution will also influence its osmotic pressure. An isotonic solution is a solution that has the same osmotic pressure as a body fluid. If the osmotic pressure is lower than body fluid, the solution is hypotonic and can cause cell lysis. Hypertonic solutions have a higher osmotic pressure than a body fluid and can cause shrinkage of red blood cells. For many routes of administration it is important that a solution is isotonic. Often sodium chloride is used to make a solution isotonic. To prepare isotonic solutions, methods that consider freezing point depression, molecular concentration, or sodium chloride equivalents can be used.

# 4.7 Answers to self-assessment questions

This section contains the worked answers for the self-assessment questions within section 4.5.

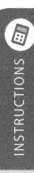

### The use of calculators for the self-assessment questions in this chapter

It is recommended that you undertake the following calculations using a calculator.

INSTRUCTIONS

**QUESTION 4.1:** *You add 5 mL of diluent to an ampoule containing 500 mg of amoxicillin. The final volume is 5.4 mL. What is the displacement value for the powder in the ampoule?*

**ANSWER:** 0.4 mL/500 mg.

**QUESTION 4.2:** *The displacement value for diamorphine as a powder for reconstitution is 0.6 mL/5 mg. What volume would 40 mg of diamorphine displace?*

**ANSWER:** 4.8 mL.

**QUESTION 4.3:** *You are required to reconstitute a 1 g vial of ceftazidime to a concentration of 100 mg/mL. The powder has a displacement value of 0.9 mL. What volume of water for injection should you add to give you a final volume of 10 mL and a concentration of 100 mg/mL?*

**ANSWER:** 9.1 mL.

**QUESTION 4.4:** *You are asked to prepare an IV injection of benzylpenicillin at 150 mg/mL. You have 600 mg vials of benzylpenicillin and the displacement value for this powder is 0.4 mL. What volume of water for injection should you add to the ampoule to achieve the required concentration?*

**ANSWER:** 3.6 mL.

**QUESTION 4.5:** *A patient requires an IV injection of meropenem at a concentration of 50 mg/mL. You have 1 g ampoules of meropenem with a displacement value of 0.9 mL. What volume of water for injection should be added to achieve the required concentration?*

**ANSWER:** 19.1 mL.

**QUESTION 4.6:** *A pharmacist receives a prescription requesting a concentration of an antibiotic suspension to be prepared to a concentration of amoxicillin 200 mg/5 mL. The label for amoxicillin powder for oral suspensions states 68 mL of water should be added to the container to give a final volume of 100 mL, with a concentration of 250 mg amoxicillin per 5 mL of suspension. What volume (in mL) should the pharmacist add to the amoxicillin powder to produce a concentration of 200 mg/5 mL?*

**ANSWER:** Addition of 68 mL will give 100 mL at a final concentration of 250 mg/5 mL.

Therefore the displacement value is 32 mL.

The total suspension requires further dilution to achieve a concentration of 200 mg/5 mL.

First calculate the total mass of drug in the container. There is 250 mg in 5 mL, therefore there is 5000 mg in 100 mL.

Next calculate the volume needed to prepare 5000 mg at 200 mg/5 mL, which is 125 mL.

Therefore the total volume required to be added is 125 mL − 32 mL = 93 mL of water is required.

Alternatively, you can calculate the additional volume required by first making up the suspension to 100 mL as per the labelling instructions, then calculating the total volume required to make the concentration 200 mg/5 mL, which is 125 mL. Therefore you add an additional 25 mL to make the total volume 125 mL.

---

**QUESTION 4.7:**  *You are required to prepare six promethazine hydrochloride suppositories, each containing 20 mg of drug and using theobroma base and 2 g nominal moulds. You prepare eight suppositories to accommodate wastage. How much drug and base do you require? The displacement value of promethazine hydrochloride is 2.5.*

**ANSWER:**  Mass of promethazine hydrochloride required = 8 × 20 mg = 160 mg.

The displacement value of promethazine hydrochloride is 2.5.

Therefore 0.16 g of promethazine hydrochloride displaces 0.064 g of base.

Total amount of base required = (8 × 2g) − 0.064 g = 15.936 g.

---

**QUESTION 4.8:**  *You are required to prepare six paracetamol suppositories, each containing 500 mg of drug and using theobroma base and 2 g nominal moulds. You prepare eight suppositories to accommodate wastage. How much drug and base do you require? The displacement value of paracetamol is 1.5.*

**ANSWER:**  Mass of paracetamol required = 8 × 500 mg = 4 g.

The displacement value of paracetamol is 1.5.

Therefore 1.5 g of paracetamol displaces 1 g of base.

Hence, 4 g of paracetamol will displace 2.67 g.

Total amount of base required = (8 × 2g) − 2.67 g = 13.33 g.

---

**QUESTION 4.9:**  *In the above preparation you change the base from theobroma oil to glycol gelatin. Assuming that a nominal 1 g mould will hold 1.2 g of glycol gelatin base, how much glycol gelatin base should be used and what will be the weight of each suppository?*

**ANSWER:**  Mass of glycol gelatin required = 1.2 ((8 × 2) − 2.67) = 16.00 g.

The total weight used = 16.00 g base + 1.2 g paracetamol = 17.20 g.

Weight per suppository = 2.15 g.

---

**QUESTION 4.10:**  *A prescription requires 150 mg miconazole nitrate pessaries prepared using a 2 g nominal mould. What would be the displacement value if it is known that six pessaries with the required miconazole nitrate added weigh 12.34 g?*

**ANSWER:**  Six pessaries without drug = 12 g.

Six pessaries with drug = 12.34 g.

Amount of drug in the pessaries = $0.15 \times 6 = 0.9$ g.

Therefore amount of base in the pessaries = $12.34 - 0.9 = 11.44$ g.

Therefore the amount of base displaced by the drug = $12 - 11.44$ g = $0.56$ g.

Therefore 0.56 g of base was displaced by 0.9 g of drug.

Therefore the displacement value is 1.6.

---

**QUESTION 4.11:** *1% w/v of chloramphenicol solution freezes at −0.06°C. What concentration of NaCl (as w/v) is required to make this solution isotonic? Note a 1% w/v of NaCl solution freezes at −0.576°C.*

**ANSWER:** An isotonic solution freezes at −0.52°C.

1% w/v of chloramphenicol solution freezes at −0.06°C.

The freezing point needs to be reduced by 0.46°C.

Therefore $-0.46 \div -0.576 = 0.80\%$ w/v of NaCl is required.

---

**QUESTION 4.12:** *1% w/v of morphine sulfate solution freezes at −0.08°C and a 1% w/v of NaCl solution freezes at −0.576°C. What concentration of NaCl (as w/v) is required to make this solution isotonic? What mass of NaCl will be required to prepare a 30 mL solution?*

**ANSWER:** An isotonic solution freezes at −0.52°C.

1% w/v of morphine sulfate solution freezes at −0.08°C.

The freezing point needs to be reduced by 0.44°C.

Therefore $-0.44 \div -0.576 = 0.76\%$ w/v of NaCl is required.

0.76% w/v NaCl = 0.76 g per 100 mL.

Therefore for 30 mL = $(0.76g \times 30) \div 100 = 0.23$ g of NaCl is required.

---

**QUESTION 4.13:** *1% w/v of glucose solution freezes at −0.091°C. What concentration of glucose (as w/v) is required to prepare an isotonic solution with a freezing point of −0.52°C?*

**ANSWER:** −0.091°C is the freezing point of 1% solution.

Therefore $-0.52 \div -0.091 = 5.7\%$ w/v of glucose solution would be isotonic.

---

**QUESTION 4.14:** *Calculate how much NaCl is required to make a 10 mL bottle of 0.5% chloramphenicol eye drops isotonic given that 1% w/v of chloramphenicol solution freezes at −0.06°C and a 1% w/v of NaCl solution freezes at −0.576°C.*

**ANSWER:** An isotonic solution freezes at −0.52°C.

1% w/v of chloramphenicol solution freezes at −0.06°C.

0.5% w/v will freeze at $0.06°C \times 0.5 = 0.03°C$.

The freezing point needs to be reduced by 0.49°C.

Therefore $-0.49 \div -0.576 = 0.85\%$ w/v of NaCl is required.

0.85% = 0.85 g in 100 mL, therefore for 10 mL, 0.085 g NaCl is required.

---

**QUESTION 4.15:** *Ephedrine sulfate injection is a sterile solution of ephedrine sulfate in water. Each mL contains 30 mg of ephedrine sulfate. How much sodium chloride is required to make this 1 mL solution isotonic given that 1% w/v of ephedrine sulfate freezes at −0.13°C and a 1% w/v of NaCl solution freezes at −0.576°C?*

| ANSWER: | An isotonic solution freezes at −0.52°C. |
|---|---|
| | 1% w/v of ephedrine freezes at −0.13°C. |
| | The solution contains 30 mg per mL, therefore 3 g in 100 mL, therefore is a 3% solution. |
| | 3% w/v will freeze at −0.13°C × 3 = −0.39°C. |
| | The freezing point needs to be reduced by 0.13°C. |
| | Therefore −0.13 ÷ −0.576 = 0.226% w/v of NaCl is required. |
| | 0.226% = 0.226 g in 100 mL, therefore for 1 mL, 0.00226 g or 2.26 mg NaCl is required. |

**QUESTION 4.16:** *What mass of dextrose is required to produce 200 mL of a solution that is isotonic with blood? The MW of dextrose is 180.*

| ANSWER: | The osmolarity of blood = 0.3 mol/L. |
|---|---|
| | Dextrose has one osmotically active species as it does not dissociate, therefore the concentration of dextrose is 0.3 mol/L. |
| | MW of dextrose is 180, therefore a 1 molar solution is 180 g/L. |
| | 0.3 M is 0.3 × 180 g/L = 54 g/L. |
| | For 200 mL, 10.8 g of dextrose is required. |

**QUESTION 4.17:** *What mass of KCl is required to produce 100 mL of a solution that is isotonic with blood? The MW of KCl = 74.5.*

| ANSWER: | The osmolarity of blood = 0.3 mol/L. |
|---|---|
| | KCl has two osmotically active species ($K^+$ and $Cl^-$), therefore the concentration of KCl is 0.15 mol/L. |
| | MW of KCl = 74.5 therefore 1 mol/L = 74.5 g/L. |
| | 0.15 M = 0.15 × 74.5 g/L = 11.175 g/L. |
| | Therefore, 100 mL requires 1.12 g. |

**QUESTION 4.18:** *What molar concentration of NaCl is required to make a 1.5% w/v dextrose solution isotonic with blood? (MW of dextrose is 180.)*

| ANSWER: | The osmolarity of blood = 0.3 mol/L. |
|---|---|
| | 1.5% w/v dextrose = 1.5 g/100 mL = 15 g/L. |
| | Molar concentration = 15 ÷ 180 = 0.08 mol/L. |
| | Dextrose has one osmotically active species, therefore dextrose solution supplies 0.08 moles/L. |
| | Thus an additional 0.22 mol/L is required to make the solution isotonic. |
| | NaCl dissociates into two active species, therefore a 0.11 molar concentration of NaCl is required. |

**QUESTION 4.19:** *How much sodium chloride is required to make a 1% w/v solution of a pilocarpine nitrate solution isotonic? (Sodium chloride equivalent of pilocarpine nitrate is 0.22.)*

| ANSWER: | The sodium chloride equivalent of pilocarpine nitrate is 0.22, that is a 1% solution of pilocarpine nitrate has the same osmotic pressure as a 0.22% solution of sodium chloride. |
|---|---|

A 0.9% NaCl solution is considered isotonic, therefore 0.68 g of sodium chloride per 100 mL of 1% solution of pilocarpine nitrate is required to make the solution isotonic.

**QUESTION 4.20:** *What mass of NaCl should be added to 80 mL of a 0.5% w/v ammonium chloride solution to make it isotonic with blood? (Sodium chloride equivalent of ammonium chloride is 1.08.)*

**ANSWER:** 1% ammonium chloride is equivalent to 1.08% NaCl.

0.5% ammonium chloride is equivalent to 0.54% NaCl.

0.9% NaCl is isotonic with blood, therefore 0.36% w/v NaCl is required.

For 100 mL this is 0.36 g, therefore for 80 mL 0.29 g NaCl is required.

**QUESTION 4.21:**

*Marcus has been prescribed 0.5 % chloramphenicol eye drugs for a bacterial eye infection. Calculate how much NaCl is required to make a 5 mL isotonic solution given 1% w/v of chloramphenicol solution freezes at −0.06°C and a 1% w/v of NaCl solution freezes at −0.576°C.*

**ANSWER:**

An isotonic solution freezes at −0.52°C.

1% w/v of chloramphenicol solution freezes at −0.06°C.

0.5% w/v will freeze at 0.06°C × 0.5 = 0.03°C.

The freezing point needs to be reduced by 0.49°C.

Therefore −0.49 ÷ −0.576 = 0.85% w/v of NaCl is required.

0.85% = 0.85 g in 100 mL, therefore for 5 mL, 42.5 mg NaCl is required.

**QUESTION 4.22:**

*Emma has been given a prescription for an oral antibiotic suspension. The label for powder for oral suspensions states 74 mL of water should be added to the container to give a final volume of 100 mL, at a concentration of 125 mg antibiotic in 5 mL. What is the displacement volume for the suspension powder and the total antibiotic content of the suspension product?*

**ANSWER:**

The volume occupied by the powder is the final volume − the volume added.

Therefore 100 mL − 74 mL = 26 mL/container content.

The concentration is 125 mg/5 mL, the total volume is 100 mL, therefore the total drug content is 2500 mg.

# Quantities to dispense: accuracy within supply

**5**

## 5.1 Chapter introduction

This chapter will cover all aspects of pharmaceutical calculations relating to the quantities of medicines to dispense in relation to different medication orders. Aspects of dispensing relating to 'special containers' will be covered in this chapter, as will the supply of medication affected by expiry of the medicinal product during the period of supply (e.g. the supply of paediatric antibiotic suspensions).

### 5.1.1 Number of days in a month

One basic question which needs to be discussed at this point is: 'how long is a month?'. Obviously a calendar month varies between 28 and 31 days, depending on the month. This causes problems with medication supply, especially repeating supply of medication for chronic illnesses, as there would need to be a range of pack sizes of pre-packed medication to cover different month lengths.

Historically, solid dosage forms (e.g. tablets and capsules) were packaged in larger 'stock' containers (e.g. 100 or 250 tablets) and so it was easy to dispense a variable quantity of medication for each administration period should this be required. However, more modern dispensing involves 'patient packs' where medication such as tablets and capsules are pre-packaged in blister strips and then put together in boxes, usually containing 28 tablets or capsules (sometimes in a single strip but often in two strips, each containing 14 dosage units). Therefore, for ease, a 'pharmaceutical month' is usually taken to be 28 days and requests for a month's supply would usually be taken to be for 28 days unless otherwise stated.

| | **EXAMPLE 5:1** |
|---|---|
| **Question:** | You are asked to supply 2 months' supply of medication where the patient has been advised to take one tablet each morning. How many tablets are required? |
| **Answer:** | In this case, there is no additional information as to the amount of medication to be supplied and so each month can be taken to be 28 days.<br><br>For 2 months' supply, we will require:<br><br>• 2 × 28 = 56 tablets.<br><br>Therefore, you need to supply 56 tablets to cover the 2-month course of medication. |

| | **EXAMPLE 5:2** |
|---|---|
| **Question:** | You are asked to supply 1 month's supply of medication where the patient has been advised to take two capsules in the morning and three in the evening. How many capsules are required? |
| **Answer:** | In this case, there is no additional information as to the amount of medication to be supplied and so each month can be taken to be 28 days.<br><br>For 1 month's supply, we will require:<br><br>• Each day, the patient will take 3 + 2 = 5 capsules.<br>• Therefore, in a pharmaceutical month they will take 5 × 28 = 140 capsules.<br><br>Therefore, you need to supply 140 capsules to cover the 1 month's course of medication. |

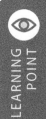

### A 'pharmaceutical month'

**LEARNING POINT**

If the quantity of medication to be supplied is in multiples of 'months', unless there is any information to the contrary, a 'pharmaceutical month' is taken to be 28 days.

Many 'patient packs' of medication are supplied in multiples of 28 (e.g. 28 tablets or 56 tablets), often containing blister strips of medication in smaller quantities (e.g. a package of 28 tablets containing two strips of 14 tablets).

### 5.1.2 Variable dosage amounts

Linked to the issue of the number of days within a calendar month potentially causing confusion as to the number of dosage units to supply to a patient, confusion can also occur when the number of dosage units to be taken at each administration varies. For example, if a patient was prescribed paracetamol tablets with a dosage instruction of 'take one or two every 4 to 6 hours' and the request was for 28 days' supply, how many tablets should we actually supply? In these cases, it is often necessary to use your professional judgement, along with information from the patient as to the likely usage of the medication. Secondly, for ease of supply and for the patient, where possible rounding the quantity to multiples of the 'patient pack' (or sub-units within the 'patient pack', e.g. one or more strips of medication) would also be sensible.

| | **EXAMPLE 5:3** |
|---|---|
| **Question:** | You are asked to supply 2 months' supply of an analgesic for a chronic condition where the patient has been advised to take: 'one or two tablets every 6 to 8 hours'. |
| **Answer:** | In this case, there is no additional information as to the amount of medication to be supplied and so each month can be taken to be 28 days. Furthermore, as the number of dosage units to be administered in each period can vary, this means that at the point of supply, the exact number of dosage units for the 2-month period is unknown.<br><br>If the patient only took one tablet at each administration point every 8 hours, we would require:<br><br>• $1 \times 3 \times 56 = 168$ tablets.<br><br>However, if the patient took two tablets at each administration point every 6 hours, we would require:<br><br>• $2 \times 4 \times 56 = 448$ tablets.<br><br>So, assuming that the patient took at least one tablet at each period at the minimum frequency (as, of course, they could take fewer), we need to supply between 168 and 448 tablets.<br><br>Upon speaking to the patient, you understand that they take, on average, around six tablets per day (they tend to take two tablets every 8 hours), although at times they take up to eight tablets a day. This would require:<br><br>• $2 \times 3 \times 56 = 336$ tablets.<br><br>If the tablets were packaged in multiples of 100, it would therefore make sense to supply $4 \times 100$. This would cover the suggested number of dosage units required based on the patient's estimation of their requirements (taking into consideration that they do at times take more than six tablets a day) and still also within the suggested range of tablets required, which was 168-448.<br><br>Therefore, in this case you should supply 400 tablets to cover the 2-month course of tablets. |

**Variable dosing**

If the number of dosage units to be administered at each point is dependent on other factors (e.g. the level of a patient's pain), then it is not immediately obvious how many dosage units to supply. In these cases, it is often useful to work out the dosage unit 'range' based on the minimum and maximum amount a patient could take. Then, with additional information from the patient or other suitable sources, a sensible amount to provide becomes more obvious.

When deciding on this final amount, it is often useful to give consideration to the pack size of the medication to ensure that wherever possible, whole multiples of the pack size (or sub-pack units) are supplied.

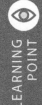

LEARNING POINT

# 5.2 Basic quantity calculations: solid dosage forms

From a calculations perspective, the supply of solid dosage forms is, in some ways, relatively straightforward. For example, if a prescriber requests supply of 28 capsules for a 1-week course of antibiotics (i.e. one to be taken four times a day for a week), it is a simple matter of supplying the 28 capsules. In relation to the number of dosage units to supply, no further calculations are required. However, in some cases, it is necessary to calculate the number of dosage units for the supply based on the quantity to be taken and the duration of the supply.

| | **EXAMPLE 5:4** |
|---|---|
| **Question:** | You are asked to supply the following course of prednisolone 5 mg tablets: |
| | • 6 OD 1/7. |
| | • 5 OD 1/7. |
| | • 4 OD 1/7. |
| | • 3 OD 1/7. |
| | • 2 OD 1/7. |
| | • 1 OD 5/7. |
| | How many tablets should you supply? |
| **Answer:** | This is a reducing dose of 5 mg prednisolone tablets. The best way to work out the total number of tablets to be supplied is to work it out on a day-by-day basis: |
| | This works out as follows: |
| | • 6 daily for 1 day = 6 tablets. |
| | • 5 daily for 1 day = 5 tablets. |
| | • 4 daily for 1 day = 4 tablets. |
| | • 3 daily for 1 day = 3 tablets. |
| | • 2 daily for 1 day = 2 tablets. |
| | • 1 daily for 5 days = 5 tablets. |
| | Therefore the total is 25 tablets. |
| | Therefore, you need to supply 25 tablets to cover the entire reducing course of the 5 mg prednisolone tablets. |

| | **EXAMPLE 5:5** |
|---|---|
| **Question:** | You are asked to supply the following course of prednisolone 5 mg tablets to cover a period of 28 days: |
| | • 6 OD 1/7. |
| | • 5 OD 1/7. |
| | • 4 OD 1/7. |
| | • 3 OD 1/7. |
| | • 2 OD 1/7. |
| | • 1 OD thereafter. |
| | How many tablets should you supply? |

| Answer: | This is a reducing dose of 5 mg prednisolone tablets. What is different from the calculation in Example 5:4 is that the final administration period is for the remaining days of the 28-day administration period. Therefore, in addition to calculating the number of tablets to be supplied for each of the days over the period of the reducing dose, it is also necessary to calculate the duration of the final phase of the reducing dose. As before, the best way to work out the total number of tablets to be supplied is to work it out on a day-by-day basis: |
|---|---|

This works out as follows:

- 6 daily for 1 day=6 tablets.
- 5 daily for 1 day=5 tablets.
- 4 daily for 1 day=4 tablets.
- 3 daily for 1 day=3 tablets.
- 2 daily for 1 day=2 tablets.
- 1 daily for the remaining number of days=$1 \times (28-5) = 23$ tablets.

Therefore the total is 43 tablets.

Therefore, you need to supply 43 tablets to cover the entire reducing course of the 5 mg prednisolone tablets.

## 5.3 Basic quantity calculations: liquid dosage forms

In many ways, the calculations relating to the supply of liquid dosage forms are the same as those for solid dosage forms. The key differences are:

(a) In many cases, an overage must be supplied to allow for any transference losses encountered during the process of measuring the dosages.

(b) Particular consideration needs to be made of any expiration dates as many liquid preparations, especially those which are reconstituted from a solid at the point of dispensing, will expire much earlier than an equivalent solid dosage form.

(c) Any supply of bulk liquid will require further manipulation by the patient or parent/guardian/carer at the point of administration.

This latter point adds a step to the administration process and so care needs to be taken at the time of supply to ensure that the dosage to be measured can be achieved easily with commercially available pharmaceutical measuring devices.

| | **EXAMPLE 5:6** |
|---|---|
| Question: | You are asked to calculate a sufficient quantity (not including an overage) for the following prescription:<br>• 5 mL to be taken four times a day for 5 days. |
| Answer: | To work out the total quantity for this supply, you need to calculate the number of individual doses required and multiply this by the volume of the dose. |

Therefore, you require:

- $4 \times 5 = 20$ doses of 5 mL per dose.
- $20 \times 5 = 100$ mL.

Therefore, you need to supply a minimum of 100 mL to cover the administration period (not taking into consideration any overage).

| | |
|---|---|
| **EXAMPLE 5:7** | |
| **Question:** | You are asked to calculate a sufficient quantity (not including an overage) for the following prescription:<br><br>• 15 mL to be taken three times a day for a week. |
| **Answer:** | To work out the total quantity for this supply, you need to calculate the number of individual doses required and multiply this by the volume of the dose.<br><br>Therefore, you require:<br><br>• $3 \times 7 = 21$ doses of 15 mL per dose.<br>• $21 \times 15 = 315$ mL.<br><br>Therefore, you need to supply a minimum of 315 mL to cover the administration period (not taking into consideration any overage). |

## 5.4 Basic quantity calculations: special containers

Special containers are containers that cannot be split. As such, you will need to supply the nearest whole number of containers to cover the amount of medication required. For example, an inhaler for the delivery of medicament to the respiratory tract would contain a number of inhalations within each canister. It is not feasible to supply these in anything other than multiples of the canister (i.e. multiples of the number of inhalations within each canister). Therefore, if each canister contains 100 inhalations, these must be supplied in multiples of 100 (i.e. 1 canister is 100 inhalations, 2 canisters are 200 inhalations, etc.).

Please note that when supplying against the receipt of an NHS prescription form, the 'rules' to follow as to whether you should round-up or round-down can be found in the respective Drug Tariff (i.e. the *Drug Tariff for England and Wales*, the *Northern Ireland Drug Tariff*, and the *Scottish Drug Tariff*). For the purpose of this book, we will assume that all calculations are undertaken to ensure that sufficient medicinal product is provided to cover the requested administration period.

| | |
|---|---|
| **EXAMPLE 5:8** | |
| **Question:** | You are asked to supply a sufficient quantity of inhalers (200 inhalations per inhaler) for the following prescription:<br><br>• Two puffs to be inhaled three times a day for 2 months. |
| **Answer:** | To work out the total quantity for this supply, you need to (a) calculate the number of individual doses required and (b) compare this with the number of inhalations in each inhaler. |

Therefore, you require:

- $2 \times 3 \times (28 \times 2)$.
- $6 \times 56 = 336$ inhalations.

Therefore, if each inhaler contains 200 inhalations, you will need to supply two inhalers to cover the administration period.

| | EXAMPLE 5:9 |
|---|---|
| Question: | You are asked to supply a sufficient quantity of cream (100 g of cream per container) for the following prescription:<br><br>&bull; Apply to both hands twice a day for 3 weeks. |
| Answer: | To work out the total quantity for this supply, you need to (a) calculate the amount of cream required for each administration and (b) multiply this by the administration period.<br><br>According to the *British National Formulary*[6] the amount of cream required for twice-daily administration to both hands for a week is:<br><br>&bull; 25-50 g.<br><br>Therefore, we will need to multiply this by three for the required administration period (of 3 weeks), giving the required amount as:<br><br>&bull; 75-150 g.<br><br>Therefore, if the cream is packaged in 100 g containers, you will need to supply one or two containers depending on the patient's usage within the application range. |

## Amounts of creams, ointments, and lotions to be supplied

If the amount of cream, ointment, or lotion to be supplied is not indicated on the prescription, in certain cases it will be necessary to estimate the amount of preparation which will be used. In section 13.1.2 of the *British National Formulary*, there is a table that provides suggested amounts of cream, ointment, or lotion for twice-daily administration for a week for the following areas:

- Both arms or both legs.
- Both hands.
- Face.
- Groin and genitalia.
- Scalp.
- Trunk.

LEARNING POINT

6 *British National Formulary* 67th Edition, Section 13.1.2, page 764.

# 5.5 Quantity calculations: intravenous infusions

Intravenous infusions provide a further set of calculations with which you need to be familiar. These calculations are based on the quantity of an infusion to be made based on the amount of drug to be administered over a specific period. Calculations in this section are relatively straightforward and relate to the quantity of medication to supply. More complex calculations involved in the supply of medication via intravenous infusions, and the infusion rate, etc., are covered in Chapter 7.

| | **EXAMPLE 5:10** |
|---|---|
| **Question:** | You are asked to supply a sufficient quantity of an infusion for the following prescription: |
| | • Prepare a 10 mg/5 mL infusion and administer 300 mg over a 2-hour period. |
| **Answer:** | To work out the total quantity of infusion to be prepared, we divide the total quantity of drug to be administered by the amount in each volume unit. |
| | In this example, there are 10 mg/5 mL of infusion and we need to administer 300 mg. Therefore, for 300 mg we will need: |
| | • $(300 \div 10) \times 5$ mL of infusion. |
| | • $30 \times 5 = 150$ mL of infusion. |
| | Therefore, we need to supply 150 mL of 10 mg/5 mL infusion and administer this over the 2-hour period. |

| | **EXAMPLE 5:11** |
|---|---|
| **Question:** | If the infusion in Example 5:10 is to be prepared from an injection that contains 100 mg in 10 mL, how many injections are required to make the infusion? |
| **Answer:** | To calculate the number of injections to use, we need to divide the total amount of drug required by the amount per injection. |
| | In this example, we require 300 mg of drug and each injection contains 100 mg in every 10 mL. Therefore, we require: |
| | • $300 \div 100 =$ three injections. |
| | Therefore, we need three injections to provide the 300 mg necessary for the infusion. In addition, the volume of the injection will occupy: |
| | • $3 \times 10$ mL $= 30$ mL (as each injection contains 100 mg in 10 mL). |
| | Therefore, to prepare 150 mL of infusion, we require three injections and: |
| | • $150 - 30 = 120$ mL of vehicle. |

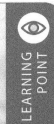

### Preparation of infusions

When preparing an infusion for administration to a patient, this is often achieved by diluting a more concentrated solution. In these cases, it is always necessary to take into consideration the volume of the more concentrated solutions and subtract this from the required final volume when calculating the amount of vehicle required.

If the injections are to be added to a pre-prepared infusion bag, it is often necessary to remove a quantity of the liquid in the bag which is equal to the amount of liquid to be added. This is because in many cases, it is not possible to add further liquid to the bag (even if the dosage calculation had allowed for this) owing to the limited available free space in the infusion bag. Therefore, calculations should be based on the original volume (or a smaller volume) of the pre-filled bag.

Finally, it is necessary to highlight that there are a number of different vehicles that can be used for infusions, and it is important to give consideration to the compatibility of the drug or drugs with the diluent. Information about compatibilities is beyond the scope of this book but information can be found in the *British National Formulary*, in specialized intravenous medication texts, and within the *Summary of Product Characteristics* supplied with each medicinal product.

Calculations involving the administration rates of intravenous infusions are covered in Chapter 7.

## 5.6 Expiration of medication during the supply period

Some medication will require reconstitution within the pharmacy before being supplied to the patient. In these cases, it is important to be aware of the expiry date of the reconstituted medication (as opposed to the expiry date of the medication before it was reconstituted, which is likely to be much longer) as it is possible with some products that the reconstituted medicament will expire before the completion of the supply period. This is particularly the case with antibiotic mixtures (often used for paediatric patients), but can also be the case for certain individual patient products such as reconstituted chemotherapeutic agents for oncology patients.

| | EXAMPLE 5:12 |
|---|---|
| **Question:** | You are asked to supply an antibiotic mixture for a 6-year-old: '2.5 mL to be given four times a day for 2 weeks'. The reconstituted medicine comes in multiples of 100 mL and expires 7 days after reconstitution. |
| **Answer:** | To work out the total quantity for this supply, you need to calculate the number of individual doses required and multiply this by the volume of the dose. Therefore, you require: <br>• $14 \times 4 = 56$ doses of 2.5 mL per dose. <br>• $56 \times 2.5 = 140$ mL. |

Therefore, you need to supply a minimum of 140 mL to cover the administration period (not taking into consideration any overage).

However, it is noted that the reconstituted medication comes in multiples of 100 mL and will expire 7 days following reconstitution.

Therefore, you will have to supply 2 × 100 mL (to cover the required 140 mL). Furthermore, this will need to be supplied in two stages; one reconstituted 100 mL now, with any remainder to be discarded after 7 days, and one reconstituted 100 mL in 7 days' time to complete the course. In addition, the supply of 100 mL for each week will take account of any overage required (as each week's supply will be for 100 mL, with a requirement of 70 mL per week).

---

**EXAMPLE 5:13**

**Question:** You are asked to supply an antibiotic mixture for a 9-month-old: '2 mL to be given three times a day for 1 week'. The reconstituted medicine comes in multiples of 50 mL and expires 7 days after reconstitution.

**Answer:** To work out the total quantity for this supply, you need to calculate the number of individual doses required and multiply this by the volume of the dose.

Therefore, you require:

- 7 × 3 = 21 doses of 2 mL per dose.
- 21 × 2 = 42 mL.

Therefore, you need to supply a minimum of 42 mL to cover the administration period (not taking into consideration any overage).

However, it is noted that the reconstituted medication comes in multiples of 50 mL and will expire 7 days following reconstitution.

Therefore, you will have to supply 1 × 50 mL (to cover the required 42 mL). Although the reconstituted product will expire in a week, this corresponds to the length of the course and so in this case, does not cause a problem (unlike in Example 5:12). In addition, the supply of 50 mL will take account of any overage required (as the total supply will be for 50 mL, with a requirement of 42 mL for the week's course).

## 5.7 Self-assessment questions

### 5.7.1 Basic self-assessment questions

This section contains a number of basic self-assessment questions for you to undertake to ensure you have an understanding of the material in this chapter. It is recommended that you undertake all of these calculations **without a calculator** and then check your answers with the answers in section 5.9.

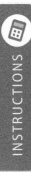

## The use of calculators for the self-assessment questions in this chapter

It is recommended that you undertake the following calculations without the use of a calculator.

All of the self-assessment questions within this section can be undertaken using a pen and paper.

INSTRUCTIONS

**QUESTION 5.1:** *You are asked to supply 3 months' supply of medication where the patient has been advised to take one tablet twice a day. How many tablets are required?*

**QUESTION 5.2:** *You are asked to supply 2 months' supply of medication where the patient has been advised to take one capsule in the morning and two in the evening. How many capsules are required?*

**QUESTION 5.3:** *You are asked to supply 1 month's supply of an analgesic for a chronic condition where the patient has been advised to take: 'one or two tablets up to four times a day'. Upon speaking to the patient, you understand that they take on average around six tablets per day (although sometimes they take fewer). The tablets are packaged in multiples of 50.*

**QUESTION 5.4:** *You are asked to supply the following course of prednisolone 5 mg tablets:*

- *6 OD 1/7.*
- *5 OD 2/7.*
- *4 OD 2/7.*
- *3 OD 2/7.*
- *2 OD 3/7.*
- *1 OD 14/7.*

*How many tablets should you supply?*

**QUESTION 5.5:** *You are asked to supply the following course of prednisolone 5 mg tablets to cover a period of 28 days:*

- *6 OD 3/7.*
- *5 OD 3/7.*
- *4 OD 3/7.*
- *3 OD 3/7.*
- *2 OD 3/7.*
- *1 OD thereafter.*

*How many tablets should you supply?*

**QUESTION 5.6:** *You are asked to calculate a sufficient quantity (not including an overage) for the following prescription:*

- *5 mL to be taken twice a day for 7 days.*

**QUESTION 5.7:** You are asked to calculate a sufficient quantity (not including an overage) for the following prescription:

• 20 mL to be taken three times a day for 2 weeks.

**QUESTION 5.8:** You are asked to supply a sufficient quantity of inhalers (100 inhalations per inhaler) for the following prescription:

• Two puffs to be inhaled twice a day for 1 month.

**QUESTION 5.9:** You are asked to supply a sufficient quantity of ointment (30 g of ointment per container) for the following prescription:

• Apply to the face daily for 4 weeks.

The British National Formulary[7] advises that for creams and ointments applied to the face, 15-30 g would be required for a week of twice-daily applications.

**QUESTION 5.10:** You are asked to supply a sufficient quantity of an infusion for the following prescription:

• Prepare a 15 mg/10 mL infusion and administer 450 mg over a 5-hour period.

**QUESTION 5.11:** If the infusion in Question 5.10 is to be prepared from an injection which contains 30 mg in 5 mL, how many injections are required to make the infusion?

**QUESTION 5.12:** You are asked to supply an antibiotic mixture for a 4-year-old patient according to the following prescription:

• 5 mL to be given three times a day for 2 weeks.

Once reconstituted, each container will contain 120 mL of liquid and will last for 7 days.

**QUESTION 5.13:** You are asked to supply an antibiotic mixture for a 3-month-old patient according to the following prescription:

• 1.25 mL to be given six times a day for 1 week.

Once reconstituted, each container will contain 20 mL of liquid and will last for 7 days.

### 5.7.2 Running case studies

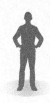

**QUESTION 5.14:**

John Jones is suffering from indigestion (which is probably linked to his love for the pub and curry house). He has been prescribed an antacid liquid, which he should take every 6 hours. The dose is 5 mL and you have been asked to supply sufficient for 2 weeks. The antacid comes in 300 mL bottles—how many should you supply to ensure that John has sufficient?

---

7 *British National Formulary* 67th Edition, Section 13.1.2, page 764.

**QUESTION 5.15:**

*Geoff cut his hand at work on a saw and following a minor procedure to help the cut heal, has been prescribed a course of analgesia. The direction on the prescription is as follows: 'Take one to two every 8 hours'. You have been asked to provide Geoff with sufficient medication for a week. On speaking to Geoff, he tells you that his injury is quite painful. The medication comes in boxes of 100, each containing 10 strips of 10 tablets. How many tablets to the nearest strip of 10 tablets should you supply?*

# 5.8 Summary

This chapter has provided a summary of the basics around the supply of the right quantity of mediation to the patient. Although in many cases the quantity of medication to supply is obvious from the medication order, other prescriptions require calculation of the quantity from administration instructions in conjunction with information about the length of time the supply is for. In some cases, for example in cases where a patient will vary the amount of medication taken in line with changes in symptoms (e.g. in the case of pain control), it is necessary to calculate a suitable quantity to supply using additional information (e.g. in consultation with the patient). It is expected that you are familiar with the concepts covered within this chapter as subsequent chapters will include the types of calculations covered.

# 5.9 Answers to self-assessment questions

This section contains the worked answers for the self-assessment questions within section 5.7.

**The use of calculators for the self-assessment questions in this chapter**

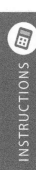

It is recommended that you undertake the following calculations without the use of a calculator.

All of the self-assessment questions within this section can be undertaken using a pen and paper.

INSTRUCTIONS

---

**QUESTION 5.1:**  *You are asked to supply 3 months' supply of medication where the patient has been advised to take one tablet twice a day. How many tablets are required?*

**ANSWER:**  In this case, there is no additional information as to the amount of medication to be supplied and so each month can be taken to be 28 days.

For 3 months' supply, we will require:

- $1 \times 2 \times (28 \times 3) = 168$ tablets.

Therefore, you need to supply 168 tablets to cover the 3-month course of medication.

**QUESTION 5.2:** *You are asked to supply 2 months' supply of medication where the patient has been advised to take one capsule in the morning and two in the evening. How many capsules are required?*

**ANSWER:** In this case, there is no additional information as to the amount of medication to be supplied and so each month can be taken to be 28 days.

For 2 months' supply, we will require:

- Each day, the patient will take $1+2=3$ capsules.
- Therefore, in a pharmaceutical month they will take $3\times28=84$ capsules.
- Therefore, in 2 months they will take $84\times2=168$.

Therefore, you need to supply 168 capsules to cover the two months' course of medication.

**QUESTION 5.3:** *You are asked to supply 1 month's supply of an analgesic for a chronic condition where the patient has been advised to take: 'one or two tablets up to four times a day'. Upon speaking to the patient, you understand that they take on average around six tablets per day (although sometimes they take fewer). The tablets are packaged in multiples of 50.*

**ANSWER:** In this case, there is no additional information as to the amount of medication to be supplied and so each month can be taken to be 28 days. Furthermore, as the number of dosage units to be administered in each period can vary, this means that at the point of supply, the exact number of dosage units for the 2-month period is unknown.

If the patient only took one tablet at each administration point (four times a day), we will require:

- $1\times4\times28=112$ tablets.

However, if the patient took two tablets at each administration point (four times a day), we will require:

- $2\times4\times28=224$ tablets.

So, assuming that the patient took at least one tablet at each period at the minimum frequency (as, of course, they could take fewer), we need to supply between 112 and 224 tablets.

However, speaking to the patient, you understand that they take on average around six tablets per day (although sometimes they take fewer). This would require:

- $6\times28=168$ tablets.

As the tablets are packaged in multiples of 50, it would therefore make sense to supply 150. This would cover the suggested number of dosage units required based on the patient's estimation of their requirements (taking into consideration that they do at times take fewer than six tablets a day) and is still also within the suggested range of tablets required, which was 112-224.

Therefore, in this case, you should supply 150 tablets to cover the 1-month's course of tablets.

**QUESTION 5.4:** *You are asked to supply the following course of prednisolone 5 mg tablets:*

- *6 OD 1/7.*
- *5 OD 2/7.*
- *4 OD 2/7.*
- *3 OD 2/7.*
- *2 OD 3/7.*
- *1 OD 14/7.*

*How many tablets should you supply?*

**ANSWER:** This is a reducing dose of 5 mg prednisolone tablets. The best way to work out the total number of tablets to be supplied is to work it out on a day-by-day basis:

This works out as follows:

- 6 daily for 1 day = 6 tablets.
- 5 daily for 2 days = 10 tablets.
- 4 daily for 2 days = 8 tablets.
- 3 daily for 2 days = 6 tablets.
- 2 daily for 3 days = 6 tablets.
- 1 daily for 14 days = 14 tablets.
- Therefore the total is 50 tablets.

Therefore, you need to supply 50 tablets to cover the entire reducing course of the 5 mg prednisolone tablets.

**QUESTION 5.5:** *You are asked to supply the following course of prednisolone 5 mg tablets to cover a period of 28 days:*

- *6 OD 3/7.*
- *5 OD 3/7.*
- *4 OD 3/7.*
- *3 OD 3/7.*
- *2 OD 3/7.*
- *1 OD thereafter.*

*How many tablets should you supply?*

**ANSWER:** This is a reducing dose of 5 mg prednisolone tablets. What is different to the calculation in Question 5.4 is that the final administration period is for the remaining days of the 28-day administration period. Therefore, in addition to calculating the number of tablets to be supplied for each of the days over the period of the reducing dose, it is also necessary to calculate the duration of the final phase of the reducing dose. As before, the best way to work out the total number of tablets to be supplied is to work it out on a day-by-day basis:

This works out as follows:

- 6 daily for 3 days = 18 tablets.
- 5 daily for 3 days = 15 tablets.
- 4 daily for 3 days = 12 tablets.
- 3 daily for 3 days = 9 tablets.
- 2 daily for 3 days = 6 tablets.
- 1 daily for the remaining number of days = 1 × (28-15) = 13 tablets.

Therefore the total is 73 tablets.

Therefore, you need to supply 73 tablets to cover the entire reducing course of the 5 mg prednisolone tablets.

---

**QUESTION 5.6:** *You are asked to calculate a sufficient quantity (not including an overage) for the following prescription:*

- *5 mL to be taken twice a day for 7 days.*

**ANSWER:** To work out the total quantity for this supply, you need to calculate the number of individual doses required and multiply this by the volume of the dose.

Therefore, you require:

- 2 × 7 = 14 doses of 5 mL per dose.
- 14 × 5 = 70 mL.

Therefore, you need to supply a minimum of 70 mL to cover the administration period (not taking into consideration any overage).

---

**QUESTION 5.7:** *You are asked to calculate a sufficient quantity (not including an overage) for the following prescription:*

- *20 mL to be taken three times a day for 2 weeks.*

**ANSWER:** To work out the total quantity for this supply, you need to calculate the number of individual doses required and multiply this by the volume of the dose.

Therefore, you require:

- 3 × 14 = 42 doses of 20 mL per dose.
- 42 × 20 = 840 mL.

Therefore, you need to supply a minimum of 840 mL to cover the administration period (not taking into consideration any overage).

---

**QUESTION 5.8:** *You are asked to supply a sufficient quantity of inhalers (100 inhalations per inhaler) for the following prescription:*

- *Two puffs to be inhaled twice a day for 1 month.*

**ANSWER:** To work out the total quantity for this supply, you need to (a) calculate the number of individual doses required and (b) compare this with the number of inhalations in each inhaler.

Therefore, you require:

- 2 × 2 × 28.
- 4 × 28 = 112 inhalations.

Therefore, if each inhaler contains 100 inhalations, you will need to supply two inhalers to cover the administration period.

---

**QUESTION 5.9:** *You are asked to supply a sufficient quantity of ointment (30 g of ointment per container) for the following prescription:*

- *Apply to the face daily for 4 weeks.*

*The* British National Formulary[8] *advises that for creams and ointments applied to the face, 15-30 g would be required for a week of twice-daily applications.*

**ANSWER:** To work out the total quantity for this supply, you need to (a) calculate the amount of ointment required for each administration, and (b) multiply this by the administration period.

According to the *British National Formulary*, the amount of ointment required for twice-daily administration to the face for a week is:

- 15-30 g.

However, as this is for daily administration, we need to halve these quantities for daily administration:

- 7.5-15 g.

Then, we will need to multiply this by four for the required administration period (of 4 weeks), giving the required amount as:

- 30-60 g.

Therefore, if the ointment is packaged in 30 g containers, you will need to supply one or two containers depending on the patient's usage within the application range.

---

**QUESTION 5.10:** *You are asked to supply a sufficient quantity of an infusion for the following prescription:*

- *Prepare a 15 mg/10 mL infusion and administer 450 mg over a 5-hour period.*

**ANSWER:** To work out the total quantity of infusion to be prepared, we divide the total quantity of drug to be administered by the amount in each volume unit.

In this example, there are 15 mg/10 mL of infusion and we need to administer 450 mg. Therefore, for 450 mg we will need:

- $(450 \div 15) \times 10$ mL of infusion.
- $30 \times 10 = 300$ mL of infusion.

Therefore, we need to supply 300 mL of 15 mg/10 mL infusion and administer this over the 5-hour period.

---

**QUESTION 5.11:** *If the infusion in Question 5.10 is to be prepared from an injection which contains 30 mg in 5 mL, how many injections are required to make the infusion?*

**ANSWER:** To calculate the number of injections to use, we need to divide the total amount of drug required by the amount per injection.

8 *British National Formulary* 67th Edition, Section 13.1.2, page 764.

In this example, we require 450 mg of drug and each injection contains 30 mg in every 5 mL. Therefore, we require:

- 450 ÷ 30 = 15 injections.

Therefore, we need 15 injections to provide the 450 mg necessary for the infusion. In addition, the volume of the injections will occupy:

- 15 × 5 mL = 75 mL (as each injection contains 30 mg in 5 mL).

Therefore, to prepare 300 mL of infusion, we require 15 injections and:

- 300 − 75 = 225 mL of vehicle.

**QUESTION 5.12:** *You are asked to supply an antibiotic mixture for a 4-year-old patient according to the following prescription:*

- *5 mL to be given three times a day for 2 weeks.*

*Once reconstituted, each container will contain 120 mL of liquid and will last for 7 days.*

**ANSWER:** To work out the total quantity for this supply, you need to calculate the number of individual doses required and multiply this by the volume of the dose.

Therefore, you require:

- 14 × 3 = 42 doses of 5 mL per dose.
- 42 × 5 = 210 mL.

Therefore, you need to supply a minimum of 210 mL to cover the administration period (not taking into consideration any overage).

However, it is noted that the reconstituted medication comes in multiples of 120 mL and will expire 7 days following reconstitution.

Therefore, you will have to supply 2 × 120 mL (to cover the required 210 mL). Furthermore, this will need to be supplied in two stages; one reconstituted 120 mL now, with any remainder to be discarded after 7 days, and one reconstituted 120 mL in 7 days' time to complete the course. In addition, the supply of 120 mL for each week will take account of any overage required (as each week's supply will be for 120 mL, with a requirement of 105 mL per week).

**QUESTION 5.13:** *You are asked to supply an antibiotic mixture for a 3-month-old patient according to the following prescription:*

- *1.25 mL to be given six times a day for 1 week.*

*Once reconstituted, each container will contain 20 mL of liquid and will last for 7 days.*

**ANSWER:** To work out the total quantity for this supply, you need to calculate the number of individual doses required and multiply this by the volume of the dose.

Therefore, you require:

- 7 × 6 = 42 doses of 1.25 mL per dose.
- 42 × 1.25 = 52.5 mL.

Therefore, you need to supply a minimum of 52.5 mL to cover the administration period (not taking into consideration any overage).

However, it is noted that the reconstituted medication comes in multiples of 20 mL and will expire 7 days following reconstitution.

Therefore, you will have to supply 3 × 20 mL (to cover the required 52.5 mL). Although the reconstituted product will expire in a week, this corresponds to the length of the course and so, in this case, does not cause a problem (unlike in Question 5.12). In addition, the supply of 60 mL will take account of any overage required (as the total supply will be for 60 mL, with a requirement of 52.5 mL for the week's course).

---

**QUESTION 5.14:**

*John Jones is suffering from indigestion (which is probably linked to his love for the pub and curry house). He has been prescribed an antacid liquid, which he should take every 6 hours. The dose is 5 mL and you have been asked to supply sufficient for 2 weeks. The antacid comes in 300 mL bottles—how many should you supply to ensure that John has sufficient?*

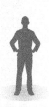

**ANSWER:**

To work out the total quantity for this supply, you need to calculate the number of individual doses required and multiply this by the volume of the dose.

Therefore, you require:

- 4 (i.e. every 6 hours) × 14 = 56 doses of 5 mL per dose.
- 56 × 5 = 280 mL.

Therefore, you need to supply a minimum of 280 mL to cover the administration period. As the medication comes in 300 mL bottles, one bottle will be sufficient to cover the administration period.

---

**QUESTION 5.15:**

*Geoff cut his hand at work on a saw and following a minor procedure to help the cut heal, has been prescribed a course of analgesia. The direction on the prescription is as follows: 'Take one to two every 8 hours'. You have been asked to provide Geoff with sufficient medication for a week. On speaking to Geoff, he tells you that his injury is quite painful. The medication comes in boxes of 100, each containing 10 strips of 10 tablets. How many tablets to the nearest strip of 10 tablets should you supply?*

**ANSWER:**

As the number of dosage units to be administered in each period can vary, this means that at the point of supply, the exact number of dosage units for the 1-week period is unknown.

If the patient only took one tablet at each administration point every 8 hours, we would require:

- $1 \times 3 \times 7 = 21$ tablets.

However, if the patient took two tablets at each administration point every 8 hours, we would require:

- $2 \times 3 \times 7 = 42$ tablets.

So, assuming that the patient took at least one tablet at each period at the minimum frequency (as, of course, they could take fewer), we need to supply between 21 and 42 tablets.

Upon speaking to the patient, you understand that the injury is quite painful and so he is likely to be taking the maximum dosage, at least for the duration of this medication supply (i.e. a week). This would require 42 tablets.

As the tablets are packaged in multiples of 100, each containing 10 strips of 10 tablets, it would therefore make sense to supply $5 \times 10$. This would cover the suggested number of dosage units required based on the patient's estimation of his requirements (and is the fewest number of strips of medication to cover this requirement).

Therefore, in this case you should supply 50 tablets to cover the 1-week course of tablets (to the nearest strip of 10 tablets).

# Handling pharmaceutical products: concentrations and dilutions

# 6

## 6.1 Chapter introduction

The ability of pharmacists and pharmacy technicians to undertake accurate calculations relating to concentrations and dilutions of pharmaceutical preparations is a key part of good pharmaceutical practice. This chapter will be set out in a number of defined sections to assist you in understanding the various mathematical manipulations involved. This will include consideration of calculations relating to percentages and ratios, concentrated and diluted solutions, and alligation. In tackling the examples and questions within this chapter, it is suggested that you familiarize yourself with the calculations covered in Chapter 2, specifically section 2.3.

## 6.2 Percentages and ratios

You will be familiar with the terms 'percentage' and 'ratio' as basic mathematical concepts. However, in pharmacy, both terms have specific meanings and when used in a pharmaceutical context, it is important you are familiar with what is meant by the specific terms.

### 6.2.1 Percentages

As outlined in section 2.3.1, percentages are used in pharmacy to express the amount of liquid or solid in a defined amount of liquid or solid. Table 6.1 recaps the terminology described in section 2.3.1.

| Term | Meaning | Example |
|---|---|---|
| **% w/w (percentage weight in weight)** | Amount of solid in grams in 100 grams of pharmaceutical product | 10% w/w = 10 g of active ingredient in every 100 g of pharmaceutical product |
| **% w/v (percentage weight in volume)** | Amount of solid in grams in 100 millilitres of pharmaceutical product | 10% w/v = 10 g of active ingredient in every 100 mL of pharmaceutical product |
| **% v/v (percentage volume in volume)** | Amount of liquid in millilitres in 100 millilitres of pharmaceutical product | 10% v/v = 10 mL of active ingredient in every 100 mL of pharmaceutical product |
| **% v/w (percentage volume in weight)** | Amount of liquid in millilitres in 100 grams of pharmaceutical product | 10% v/w = 10 mL of active ingredient in every 100 g of pharmaceutical product |

**Table 6.1** A summary of the percentage terms commonly encountered in pharmaceutical practice (from section 2.3.1)

|  | **EXAMPLE 6:1** |
|---|---|
| **Question:** | You are asked to make 630 mL of pharmaceutical product which contains 0.75% w/v of Drug A. How much active ingredient is required? |
| **Answer:** | If the final pharmaceutical product contains 0.75% w/v, this means that there is 0.75 g (or 750 mg) in every 100 mL of the product. Therefore, in 630 mL of product, there would be:<br><br>$(0.75 \div 100) \times 630 = 4.725$ g.<br><br>Therefore, you will need 4.725 g of Drug A to make 630 mL of a 0.75% w/v pharmaceutical product. |

However, in pharmacy is it often the case that we are required to produce a product from other more or less concentrated products (rather than from the pure ingredient and an inert vehicle). The conversion of concentrated liquid solutions into more dilute solutions will be covered in section 6.4. The equivalent calculations where pharmaceutical products of a particular strength are compounded from other products of different concentration (e.g. the preparation of a cream of a particular strength from a more concentrated and a more dilute cream) are termed 'alligation' and will be covered in section 6.5.

### 6.2.2 Ratios

In addition to the use of percentages in description of drug concentration, ratios are often used to express the amount of one pharmaceutical ingredient to be used relative to the amount of another. In using ratios, it is important to understand the difference between the use of the word 'to' and the word 'in'. The difference between these terms is explained in Table 6.2.

| Ratio term | Example usage | Meaning |
|---|---|---|
| 'to' | 1 to 10 (or 1:10) | One part of solute to 10 parts of solvent |
| 'in' | 1 in 10 | One part of solute in 10 parts of solvent |

**Table 6.2** The difference between 'in' and 'to' in relation to pharmaceutical ratios

| **EXAMPLE 6:2** | |
|---|---|
| **Question:** | You are required to make 210 mL of a 1 to 20 solution of Drug B (a liquid). How much Drug B is required? |
| **Answer:** | If the final pharmaceutical product contains 1 to 20 of Drug B, this means that there is 1 mL of Drug B to every 20 mL of solvent (i.e. 1 mL of Drug B in every 21 mL of product). Therefore, in 210 mL of product, there would be: $$(210 \div 21) = 10 \text{ mL}.$$ Therefore, you require 10 mL of Drug B, diluted with 200 mL (210 mL - 10 mL) of solvent to make 210 mL of a 1 to 20 solution. |

| **EXAMPLE 6:3** | |
|---|---|
| **Question:** | You are required to make 500 mL of a 1 in 25 solution of Drug C (a liquid). How much Drug C is required? |
| **Answer:** | If the final pharmaceutical product contains 1 in 25 of Drug C, this means that there is 1 mL of Drug C in every 25 mL of product. Therefore, in 500 mL of product, there would be: $$(500 \div 25) = 20 \text{ mL}.$$ Therefore, you require 20 mL of Drug C, diluted with 480 mL (500 mL − 20 mL) of solvent to make 500 mL of a 1 in 25 solution. |

## Ratios—the terms 'to' and 'in'

It is important to understand the difference between the usage of the word 'to' and 'in' when referring to ratios in pharmaceutical calculations. For example:

- 1 to 10 (or 1:10)—one part of solute to 10 parts of solvent.
- 1 in 10—one part of solute in 10 parts of solvent.

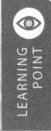

LEARNING POINT

### 6.2.3 Conversions between percentages and ratios

Later in this chapter, we will be examining how you can convert pharmaceutical preparations from one strength to another. At times, it may be that different ingredients express their concentrations in different ways and to make the subsequent calculations easier, it is necessary to convert to one format, usually percentages. Consider the following examples.

| EXAMPLE 6:4 | |
|---|---|
| **Question:** | What is the concentration of a product in percentage which contains Drug D in a concentration of 1 in 25? |
| **Answer:** | If the concentration of Drug D in the preparation is 1 in 25, this means that there is 1 part of drug for every 25 parts of product. Therefore, to convert to a percentage, we need to work out the quantity of Drug D (in mL or g) in 100 mL or g of product.<br><br>$$(1 \div 25) \times 100 = 4.$$<br><br>Therefore, a 1 in 25 product is the same as a 4% product. |

| EXAMPLE 6:5 | |
|---|---|
| **Question:** | Drug E, a liquid, is dissolved in water producing a 1 to 19 solution. What is the equivalent strength expressed as % v/v? |
| **Answer:** | If the concentration of Drug E in the preparation is 1 to 19, this means that there is 1 mL of drug to every 19 mL of water (i.e. a total of 20 mL). Therefore, to convert to a percentage (v/v), we need to work out the quantity of Drug C (in mL) in 100 mL of product.<br><br>$$(1 \div 20) \times 100 = 5.$$<br><br>Therefore, a 1 to 19 product is the same as a 5% v/v product. |

## 6.3 Preparing concentrated solutions

Before we cover the calculations involved in the preparation of solutions of certain concentrations from those of other concentrations (see section 6.4), it is necessary to understand how to prepare concentrated solutions from base ingredients. Consider the following examples; in both of these examples a particular strength of solution is prepared from a base ingredient dissolved in a particular solvent (the vehicle).

| EXAMPLE 6:6 | |
|---|---|
| **Question:** | You are required to make 3 L of a 45% w/v solution of Drug F. How much active ingredient is required? |
| **Answer:** | If the final pharmaceutical product contains 45% w/v, this means that there are 45 g in every 100 mL of the product. Therefore, in 3000 mL (3 L) of product, there would be:<br><br>$$(45 \div 100) \times 3000 = 1350\,g \equiv 1.35\,kg.$$<br><br>Therefore, you require 1.35 kg of Drug F to make 3 L of a 45% w/v solution. |

| EXAMPLE 6:7 | |
|---|---|
| **Question:** | You are required to make 700 mL of a 7.5% w/v solution of Drug G (a solid). How much active ingredient is required? |

| Answer: | If the final pharmaceutical product contains 7.5% w/v, this means that there are 7.5 g in every 100 mL of the product. Therefore, in 700 mL of product, there would be: |

$$(7.5 \div 100) \times 700 = 52.5 \, g.$$

Therefore, you require 52.5 g of Drug G to make 700 mL of a 7.5% w/v solution.

There may be times when the concentration of the solution to be prepared is at the limit or beyond the limit of an ingredient's solubility in a particular vehicle. In these cases, it is necessary to consider alternative vehicles to accommodate the quantity of solute required. If you believe that this might be the case, it is necessary to investigate the solubility of the ingredient(s) in question using suitable reference sources.

In pharmacy, the solubility of certain ingredients in particular vehicles can be found in a number of different sources, including:

- *The British Pharmacopoeia*.
- *Martindale: The Complete Drug Reference*.

| | **EXAMPLE 6:8** |
| --- | --- |
| Question: | You are required to make 200 mL of a 15% w/v solution of Sodium Bicarbonate BP in water. How much active ingredient is required? |
| Answer: | If the final pharmaceutical product contains 15% w/v, this means that there are 15 g in every 100 mL of product. Therefore, in 200 mL of product, there would be: |

$$(15 \div 100) \times 200 = 30 \, g.$$

Therefore, you would require 30 g of Sodium Bicarbonate BP to make 200 mL of a 15% w/v solution.

However, upon examining the solubility of Sodium Bicarbonate BP within the *British Pharmacopoeia*, you find that the solubility in water is 1 in 11. This means that 11 mL of vehicle is required to dissolve 1 g of Sodium Bicarbonate BP. Therefore, to dissolve your 30 g of Sodium Bicarbonate BP (the amount required for 200 mL of a 15% w/v solution), you would need:

$$30 \times 11 = 330 \, mL \text{ of water.}$$

However, 330 mL is greater than the 200 mL of vehicle required for the solution. Therefore, in this case it is not possible to make a 15% w/v solution of Sodium Bicarbonate BP in water. Depending on the reason for the original request, the options would be to make a less concentrated solution in water (and to administer a greater volume to achieve the desired quantity of Sodium Bicarbonate BP) or to research an alternative vehicle that would allow dissolution of a greater quantity of sodium bicarbonate per fixed volume.

## 6.4 Diluting solutions

Often, it is the case that the required concentration of solution is not readily available off-the-shelf. In addition, it may not be a simple matter of making the required concentration of solution from the base ingredient(s), as described in section 6.3, as the base ingredient(s) may not be readily available. In this case, it is necessary to dilute an existing solution with a greater concentration than the final solution required.

For these types of calculation, it is necessary to work out the amount of a more concentrated solution that is required to be diluted to the final volume of the required final strength. In these situations, we use the following formula:

$$C_1 V_1 = C_2 V_2$$

In this formula, the following are denoted by the symbols:

- $C_1$—this is the concentration of the original solution.
- $V_1$—this is the volume of the original solution.
- $C_2$—this is the concentration of the desired solution.
- $V_2$—this is the volume of the desired solution.

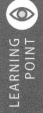

## Making dilute solutions from more concentrated solutions

For these types of calculation, it is necessary to work out the amount of a more concentrated solution that is required to be diluted to the final volume of the required final strength. In these situations, we use the following formula:

$$C_1 V_1 = C_2 V_2$$

In this formula, the following are denoted by the symbols:

- $C_1$—this is the concentration of the original solution.
- $V_1$—this is the volume of the original solution.
- $C_2$—this is the concentration of the desired solution.
- $V_2$—this is the volume of the desired solution.

LEARNING POINT

| | EXAMPLE 6:9 |
|---|---|
| **Question:** | You are required to make 450 mL of a 5% w/v solution of Drug H from a 10% solution. How much of the concentrated solution is required? |
| **Answer:** | In this situation, where we are making a particular volume of a solution from a more concentrated solution, we can use the following formula:<br><br>$$C_1 V_1 = C_2 V_2$$<br><br>In this particular case, the following values apply:<br><br> • $C_1 = 10\%$.<br> • $V_1 = $ Unknown.<br> • $C_2 = 5\%$.<br> • $V_2 = 450$ mL.<br><br>Therefore, entering the values into the equation, you get:<br><br>$10 \times V_1 = 5 \times 450$.<br>$10 \times V_1 = 2250$. |

$V_1 = 2250 \div 10$.

$V_1 = 225\,mL$.

Therefore, you will require 225 mL of a 10% solution of Drug H to make 450 mL of a 5% solution.

**EXAMPLE 6:10**

**Question:** You are told that 300 mL of a 15% w/v solution of Drug I was used to make 750 mL of a final solution. What is the concentration of this final solution?

**Answer:** Where we are making a particular volume of a solution from a more concentrated solution, we can use the following formula:

$C_1V_1 = C_2V_2$

In this particular case, the following values apply:

- $C_1 = 15\%$.
- $V_1 = 300\,mL$.
- $C_2 = $ Unknown.
- $V_2 = 750\,mL$.

Therefore, entering the values into the equation, you get:

$15 \times 300 = C_2 \times 750$.

$4500 = C_2 \times 750$.

$C_2 = 4500 \div 750$.

$C_2 = 6\%$.

Therefore, you will produce a 6% solution by diluting 300 mL of a 15% solution of Drug I to 750 mL.

**EXAMPLE 6:11**

**Question:** You are required to make 600 mL of a 3% w/v solution of Drug J from a 60% solution. How much of the concentrated solution is required?

**Answer:** Where we are making a particular volume of a solution from a more concentrated solution, we can use the following formula:

$C_1V_1 = C_2V_2$

In this particular case, the following values apply:

- $C_1 = 60\%$.
- $V_1 = $ Unknown.
- $C_2 = 3\%$.
- $V_2 = 600\,mL$.

Therefore, entering the values into the equation, you get:

$60 \times V_1 = 3 \times 600$.

$60 \times V_1 = 1800$.

$V_1 = 1800 \div 60$.

$V_1 = 30\,mL$.

Therefore, you will require 30 mL of a 60% solution of Drug J to make 600 mL of a 3% solution.

As discussed in section 1.3.2, it is always worth checking any answers you obtain by working through the answer, rather than simply re-calculating the answer again (as any calculation errors that may have been made the first time, may simply be repeated if the calculation is repeated).

In the answer to this question, we said that we would require 30 mL of a 60% solution of Drug J to make 600 mL of a 3% solution.

In 30 mL of a 60% solution, we would have:

60% is 60 g or 60 mL in 100 mL.

$(60 \div 100) \times 30 = 18\,g$ (or 18 mL).

18 g (or 18 mL) in 600 mL would produce:

$(18 \div 600) \times 100 = 3\%$.

Therefore, 30 mL of a 60% solution does make 600 mL of a 3% solution.

# 6.5 Alligation

Section 6.4 described the situation where you can calculate the required amounts of a solution and additional vehicle to make a more dilute solution. However, there will be circumstances where the only way to produce a product of the desired strength is to mix two preparations of differing concentrations (where one is of greater and one is of lesser concentration than the desired concentration). This situation is commonly encountered where there is no ready access to either the base ingredient and/or the vehicle in question (or suitable substitute vehicle), and there is a supply of products at differing concentrations. In these situations, we use a technique called alligation.

With alligation, it is important to understand that the initial calculation works out the ratio of the two products (of different concentration) to be mixed together. Once this has been established, the exact quantities for the amount of final preparation required can be calculated.

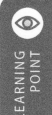

**LEARNING POINT**

**Alligation**

Alligation is used when a particular concentration of a pharmaceutical product is made by mixing two products of differing concentration; one at a higher and one at a lower concentration than the desired concentration. The alligation calculation provides the ratio of each product to be mixed together.

### 6.5.1 The alligation grid

To calculate the ratio of the two different strength ingredients to be mixed, we use the alligation grid. This is shown in Figure 6.1.

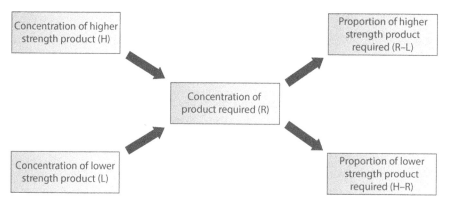

**Figure 6.1** The alligation grid.

Once you have the proportions of the individual ingredients required, you can calculate the amount of each ingredient required for your specific product.

| | EXAMPLE 6:12 |
|---|---|
| **Question:** | You are asked to produce 175 g of a 3% cream using stock creams of 5% and 1.5%. How much of each stock cream will you require? |
| **Answer:** | As this question asks for a particular strength of a product to be made, from two other products, one of a higher strength and one of a lower strength, you need to use the alligation grid (Figure 6.1) to calculate the required proportions of each ingredient.<br><br>In this particular case, the following values are calculated:<br><br>• Proportion of higher strength product required = 3 − 1.5 = 1.5.<br>• Proportion of lower strength product required = 5 − 3 = 2.<br>• Therefore, the ratio of higher strength to lower strength is 1.5 to 2.<br><br>Then, to calculate the quantity of each ingredient, we need to work out the weight of each part. In total, we require 3.5 parts (1.5 + 2) and a total weight of 175 g.<br><br>Therefore, each part weighs 175 ÷ 3.5 = 50 g.<br><br>This means that the quantity of the two products to be mixed would be:<br><br>Quantity of higher strength product = 1.5 × 50 = 75 g.<br><br>Quantity of lower strength product = 2 × 50 = 100 g.<br><br>Therefore, you need to mix 75 g of 5% cream with 100 g of 1.5% cream to produce 175 g of 3% cream. |

As discussed in section 1.3.2 it is useful to be able to self-check calculations, especially if the calculated answer is not obviously correct. In Example 6:12, the first check to undertake would be to make sure that the calculated proportions add up to the required total weight. In this case, 75 g and 100 g, they do total the required final weight of cream (175 g). However, it is not immediately obvious that the two quantities of the different strength creams, once combined, will in fact produce a cream of the desired strength. Example 6:13 demonstrates how you can check the values.

| **EXAMPLE 6:13** | |
|---|---|
| **Question:** | In Example 6:12, we calculated that 75 g of 5% cream mixed with 100 g of 1.5% cream would produce 175 g of 3% cream. |
| **Answer:** | To check this calculation, we need to calculate the amount of actual drug each cream would contribute to the final product, and then work out the resultant strength of the final product.<br><br>The higher strength product contains the active ingredient at 5% strength. This means that there are 5 g (or mL) of active ingredient per 100 g. If we are using 75 g of this product, there will be:<br><br>• $(5 \div 100) \times 75 = 3.75$ g (or mL).<br><br>The lower strength product contains the active ingredient at 1.5% strength. This means that there are 1.5 g (or mL) of active ingredient per 100 g. If we are using 100 g of this product, there will be:<br><br>• $(1.5 \div 100) \times 100 = 1.5$ g (or mL).<br><br>Therefore, in the total 175 g of product, there will be:<br><br>• $3.75 + 1.5 = 5.25$ g (or mL) of active ingredient.<br><br>This will produce a product of the following strength:<br><br>• $(5.25 \div 175) \times 100 = 3\%$.<br><br>As 3% was the desired strength, it means that the calculation in Example 6:12 is correct. |

In Example 6:12, the question asked how much of two different ingredients are required to produce a stated quantity of a different strength preparation. In giving the answer, it is possible to state the quantity of each of the two ingredients to be mixed to obtain the final product. The other type of calculation in which alligation can be used is where more active ingredient is added to a particular strength and quantity of a product to produce a higher strength.

| **EXAMPLE 6:14** | |
|---|---|
| **Question:** | You are asked to produce 480 g of a 6% cream using stock cream of 4% and the active ingredient. How much of the stock cream and the active ingredient will you require? |
| **Answer:** | This question is similar to Example 6:12 in that one of the two items to be mixed together is pure ingredient and can be taken as having a concentration of 100%. Therefore, as before, we can use the alligation grid (Figure 6.1) to calculate the required proportions of each ingredient.<br><br>In this particular case, the following values are calculated:<br><br>• Proportion of higher strength product required = $6 - 4 = 2$.<br><br>• Proportion of lower strength product required = $100 - 6 = 94$.<br><br>• Therefore, the ratio of higher strength to lower strength is 2 to 94. |

Then, to calculate the quantity of each ingredient, we need to work out the weight of each part. In total, we require 96 parts (2 + 94) and a total weight of 480 g.

Therefore, each part weighs 480 ÷ 96 = 5 g.

This means that the quantity of the two products to be mixed would be:

Quantity of active ingredient = 2 × 5 = 10 g.

Quantity of lower strength product = 94 × 5 = 470 g.

Therefore, you need to mix 470 g of 4% cream with 10 g of active ingredient to produce 480 g of 6% cream.

As with Example 6:12, it is useful to check the calculated values using the alligation grid. The first check to make would be that the calculated proportions add up to the required total weight. In this case, 10 g and 470 g, they do total the required final weight of cream (480 g). However, as with Example 6:12, it is not immediately obvious that the two quantities (in this case of the lower strength cream and the active ingredient) once combined will produce a cream of the desired strength. Example 6:15 demonstrates how you can check the values.

| | **EXAMPLE 6:15** |
|---|---|
| **Question:** | In Example 6:14, we calculated that 470 g of 4% cream mixed with 10 g of active ingredient would produce 480 g of 6% cream. |
| **Answer:** | To check this calculation, we need to calculate the amount of actual drug each ingredient would contribute to the final product, and then work out the resultant strength of the final product. |

The higher strength product contains pure active ingredient (i.e. 100%). This means that there are 10 g of active ingredient being added to the lower strength cream.

The lower strength product contains the active ingredient at 4% strength. This means that there are 4 g of active ingredient per 100 g. If we are using 470 g of this product, there will be:

- $(4 \div 100) \times 470 = 18.8$ g.

Therefore, in the total 480 g of product, there will be:

- $10 + 18.8 = 28.8$ g of active ingredient.

This will produce a product of the following strength:

- $(28.8 \div 480) \times 100 = 6\%$.

As 6% was the desired strength, it means that the calculation in Example 6:14 is correct.

Next, we examine the same style of calculation but one in which the proportions do not relate as easily to the quantity of cream required (i.e. parts of the calculation will necessitate the answer(s) being stated to a number of decimal places).

| | **EXAMPLE 6:16** |
|---|---|
| **Question:** | You are asked to produce 500 g of a 9.5% cream using stock cream of 1% and the active ingredient. How much of the stock cream and the active ingredient (each to two decimal places) will you require? |
| **Answer:** | This question is similar to Example 6:14 in that one of the two items to be mixed together is pure ingredient and can be taken as having a concentration of 100%. Therefore, as before, we can use the alligation grid (Figure 6.1) to calculate the required proportions of each ingredient. |

In this particular case, the following values are calculated:

- Proportion of higher strength product required $= 9.5 - 1 = 8.5$.
- Proportion of lower strength product required $= 100 - 9.5 = 90.5$.
- Therefore, the ratio of higher strength to lower strength is 8.5 to 90.5.

Then, to calculate the quantity of each ingredient, we need to work out the weight of each part. In total, we require 99 parts (8.5 + 90.5) and a total weight of 500 g.

Therefore, each part weighs $500 \div 99 = 5.05$ g (to two decimal places).

This means that the quantity of the two products to be mixed would be:

Quantity of active ingredient $= 8.5 \times (500 \div 99) = 42.93$ g (to two decimal places).

Quantity of lower strength product $= 90.5 \times (500 \div 99) = 457.07$ g (to two decimal places).

Therefore, you need to mix 457.07 g of 1% cream with 42.93 g of active ingredient to produce 500 g of 9.5% cream.

**The use of decimal places in calculations**

In Example 6:16, you will notice that in the two calculations relating to the quantity of each of the individual ingredients to be combined, the value of each part was left as the fraction (500 ÷ 99), rather than the absolute value as demonstrated in Example 6:14. This was to reduce the error that could have been caused by successive rounding. Wherever possible, reduce the number of times you round values in the calculation process, reserving rounding to the final answer wherever possible.

LEARNING POINT

As demonstrated in Example 6:15 (relating to Example 6:14), it is useful to check the values you have calculated using the alligation grid and the first check to make would be that the calculated proportions add up to the required total weight. This is especially important in this example as the proportions of the two ingredients to be combined do not relate as easily to the quantity of cream required (as they did in Example 6:15). In this case, 42.93 g and 457.07 g, they do total the required final weight of cream (500 g). However, as with Example 6:15, it is not immediately obvious that the two quantities (the lower strength cream and the active ingredient) once combined will produce a cream of the desired strength. Example 6:17 demonstrates how you can check the values.

| | **EXAMPLE 6:17** |
|---|---|
| **Question:** | In Example 6:16, we calculated that 457.07 g of 1% cream mixed with 42.93 g of active ingredient would produce 500 g of 9.5% cream. |
| **Answer:** | To check this calculation, we need to calculate the amount of actual drug each ingredient would contribute to the final product, and then work out the resultant strength of the final product. |

The higher strength product contains pure active ingredient (i.e. 100%). This means that there are 42.93 g of active ingredient being added to the lower strength cream.

The lower strength product contains the active ingredient at 1% strength. This means that there is 1 g of active ingredient per 100 g. If we are using 457.07 g of this product, there will be:

- $(1 \div 100) \times 457.07 = 4.57$ g (to two decimal places).

Therefore, in the total 500 g of product, there will be:

- $42.93 + 4.57 = 47.5$ g of active ingredient.

This will produce a product of the following strength:

- $(47.5 \div 500) \times 100 = 9.5\%$.

As 9.5% was the desired strength, it means that the calculation in Example 6:16 is correct.

# 6.6 Self-assessment questions

## 6.6.1 Basic self-assessment questions

This section contains a number of basic self-assessment questions for you to undertake to ensure that you have an understanding of the material in this chapter. It is recommended that you undertake all of these calculations **without a calculator** and then check your answers with the answers in section 6.8.

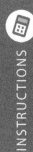

**The use of calculators for the self-assessment questions in this chapter**

It is recommended that you undertake the following calculations without the use of a calculator.

All of the self-assessment questions within this section can be undertaken using a pen and paper.

INSTRUCTIONS

**QUESTION 6.1:**  *How many grams of active ingredient are in 350 mL of a 4.7% w/v solution?*

**QUESTION 6.2:**  *How many litres of active ingredient are in 258 mL of a 10.2% v/v solution?*

**QUESTION 6.3:**  *You are required to make 910 mL of a 1 to 25 solution of Drug A (a liquid). How much Drug A is required?*

**QUESTION 6.4:**   You are required to make 420 mL of a 1 in 7 solution of Drug B (a liquid). How much Drug B is required?

**QUESTION 6.5:**   What is the concentration of a solution in percentage (to two decimal places) which contains Drug C (a solid) in a concentration of 1 in 15?

**QUESTION 6.6:**   Drug D, a liquid, is dissolved in water producing a 1 to 24 solution. What is the equivalent strength expressed as % v/v?

**QUESTION 6.7:**   You are required to make 350 mL of a 12% w/v solution of Drug E. How much active ingredient is required?

**QUESTION 6.8:**   You are required to make 25 mL of a 3.2% w/v solution of Drug F. How much active ingredient is required?

**QUESTION 6.9:**   What is the highest concentration, to the nearest whole percentage (w/v) of a solution of Sodium Bicarbonate BP in water? (Note: the solubility of Sodium Bicarbonate BP in water is stated in the British Pharmacopoeia as 1 in 11.)

**QUESTION 6.10:**   You are required to make 35 mL of a 7% w/v solution of Drug G (a solid) from a 25% solution. How much of the concentrated solution is required?

**QUESTION 6.11:**   Check the answer you obtained for Question 6.10 by working through the calculation as described in Example 6:11.

**QUESTION 6.12:**   You are told that 360 mL of a 12% w/v solution of Drug H was used to make 1 L of a final solution. What is the concentration of this final solution?

**QUESTION 6.13:**   You are required to make 2.3 L of a 6.5% w/v solution of Drug I from a 16% solution. How much of the concentrated solution is required? Once calculated, check the answer by working through the calculation as described in Example 6:11.

**QUESTION 6.14:**   You are asked to produce 350 g of a 4.6% cream using stock creams of 10% and 3%. How much of each stock cream will you require?

**QUESTION 6.15:**   Check the answer you obtained for Question 6.14 by working through the calculation as described in Example 6:13.

**QUESTION 6.16:**   You are asked to produce 75 g of a 13.5% cream using stock cream of 5.5% and the active ingredient. How much of the stock cream and the active ingredient (each to two decimal places) will you require?

**QUESTION 6.17:**   Check the answer you obtained for Question 6.16 by working through the calculation as described in Example 6:17.

### 6.6.2 Running case studies

**QUESTION 6.18:**

Evie Jones has a skin complaint and the doctor has prescribed a cream at a strength of 3.5%. The only products available have percentages of 1% and 4.5%. The doctor has requested a supply of 120 g. How much of each cream needs to be mixed together to produce 120 g at the desired strength?

**QUESTION 6.19:**

*Emma requires a solution every 6 hours to control her asthma. The dose of the drug is 5 mg/kg, four times a day. You are required to produce sufficient solution for 5 days' supply to allow each dose to be 10 mL using a 30% w/v stock solution. What quantity of stock solution is required?*

## 6.7 Summary

This chapter has provided examples and self-assessment questions around the area of pharmaceutical concentrations and dilutions. At times, it is a simple matter of calculating the required quantity of the base ingredient and a suitable vehicle to produce the desired concentration of product. However, it is also important that you are able to calculate the quantities required in the preparation of dilute solutions from more concentrated solutions, and the quantities required of two different strength preparations to produce a preparation with the desired strength in between the two (these latter calculations are termed 'alligation'). In addition, further development of the habit of self-checking introduced in Chapter 1 has been encouraged with explanation of methods for the self-checking of these more complicated calculations.

## 6.8 Answers to self-assessment questions

This section contains the worked answers for the self-assessment questions within section 6.6.

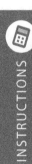

**The use of calculators for the self-assessment questions in this chapter**

It is recommended that you undertake the following calculations without the use of a calculator.

All of the self-assessment questions within this section can be undertaken using a pen and paper.

INSTRUCTIONS

---

**QUESTION 6.1:** *How many grams of active ingredient are in 350 mL of a 4.7% w/v solution?*

**ANSWER:** A 4.7% w/v solution contains 4.7 g of solid dissolved in every 100 mL of solution. Therefore, in 350 mL there would be:

$$(4.7 \div 100) \times 350 = 16.45 \, g$$

Therefore, there are 16.45 g of solid dissolved in 350 mL of a 4.7% w/v solution.

---

**QUESTION 6.2:** *How many litres of active ingredient are in 258 mL of a 10.2% v/v solution?*

**ANSWER:** A 10.2% v/v solution contains 10.2 mL of liquid dissolved in every 100 mL of solution. Therefore, in 258 mL there would be:

$$(10.2 \div 100) \times 258 = 26.316 \, mL.$$

Therefore, there are 26.316 mL of liquid dissolved in 258 mL of a 10.2% v/v solution. However, as the question asked for the answer in litres, we need to divide by 1000.

$$26.316 \div 1000 = 0.026\,316\,L.$$

Therefore, there is 0.026 316 L of liquid dissolved in 258 mL of a 10.2% v/v solution (although from a pharmaceutical perspective, it would be best to quote this figure in mL to reduce the possibility of error).

---

**QUESTION 6.3:**    *You are required to make 910 mL of a 1 to 25 solution of Drug A (a liquid). How much Drug A is required?*

**ANSWER:**    If the final pharmaceutical product contains 1 to 25 of Drug A, this means that there is 1 mL of Drug A to every 25 mL of solvent (i.e. 1 mL of Drug A in every 26 mL of product). Therefore, in 910 mL of product, there would be:

$$(910 \div 26) = 35\,mL.$$

Therefore, you require 35 mL of Drug A, diluted with 875 mL (910 − 35 mL) of solvent to make 910 mL of a 1 to 25 solution.

---

**QUESTION 6.4:**    *You are required to make 420 mL of a 1 in 7 solution of Drug B (a liquid). How much Drug B is required?*

**ANSWER:**    If the final pharmaceutical product contains 1 in 7 of Drug B, this means that there is 1 mL of Drug B in every 7 mL of product. Therefore, in 420 mL of product, there would be:

$$(420 \div 7) = 60\,mL.$$

Therefore, you require 60 mL of Drug B, diluted with 360 mL (420 − 60 mL) of solvent to make 420 mL of a 1 in 7 solution.

---

**QUESTION 6.5:**    *What is the concentration of a solution in percentage (to two decimal places) which contains Drug C (a solid) in a concentration of 1 in 15?*

**ANSWER:**    If the concentration of Drug C in the preparation is 1 in 15, this means that there is 1 part of drug for every 15 parts of product. Therefore, to convert to a percentage (w/v), we need to work out the quantity of Drug C (in g) in 100 mL of product.

$$(1 \div 15) \times 100 = 6.67 \text{ (to two decimal places)}.$$

Therefore, a 1 in 15 product is the same as a 6.67% product (to two decimal places).

---

**QUESTION 6.6:**    *Drug D, a liquid, is dissolved in water producing a 1 to 24 solution. What is the equivalent strength expressed as % v/v?*

**ANSWER:**    If the concentration of Drug D in the preparation is 1 to 24, this means that there is 1 mL of drug to every 24 mL of water (i.e. a total of 25 mL). Therefore, to convert to a percentage (v/v), we need to work out the quantity of Drug C (in mL) in 100 mL of product.

$$(1 \div 25) \times 100 = 4.$$

Therefore, a 1 to 24 product is the same as a 4% v/v product.

---

**QUESTION 6.7:**    *You are required to make 350 mL of a 12% w/v solution of Drug E. How much active ingredient is required?*

**ANSWER:**   If the final pharmaceutical product contains 12% w/v, this means that there are 12 g in every 100 mL of the product. Therefore, in 350 mL of product, there would be:

$$(12 \div 100) \times 350 = 42 \, g.$$

Therefore, you require 42 g of Drug E to make 350 mL of a 12% w/v solution.

---

**QUESTION 6.8:**   *You are required to make 25 mL of a 3.2% w/v solution of Drug F. How much active ingredient is required?*

**ANSWER:**   If the final pharmaceutical product contains 3.2% w/v, this means that there are 3.2 g in every 100 mL of the product. Therefore, in 25 mL of product, there would be:

$$(3.2 \div 100) \times 25 = 0.8 \, g \equiv 800 \, mg.$$

Therefore, you require 800 mg (0.8 g) of Drug F to make 25 mL of a 3.2% w/v solution.

---

**QUESTION 6.9:**   *What is the highest concentration, to the nearest whole percentage (w/v) of a solution of Sodium Bicarbonate BP in water? (Note: the solubility of Sodium Bicarbonate BP in water is stated in the* British Pharmacopoeia *as 1 in 11.)*

**ANSWER:**   If we want to work out the highest percentage possible, we need to calculate the number of grams of Sodium Bicarbonate BP which can be dissolved in 100 mL of water. If the solubility of Sodium Bicarbonate BP is 1 in 11, this means that 11 mL of water is required to dissolve 1 g of Sodium Bicarbonate BP. Therefore, in 100 mL, we would be able to dissolve:

$$(100 \div 11) = 9.09 \, g \text{ (to two decimal places).}$$

Therefore, to the nearest percentage, you would be able to dissolve 9 g of Sodium Bicarbonate BP in 100 mL of water. This would produce a 9% w/v solution.

---

**QUESTION 6.10:**   *You are required to make 35 mL of a 7% w/v solution of Drug G (a solid) from a 25% solution. How much of the concentrated solution is required?*

**ANSWER:**   In this situation, where we are making a particular volume of a solution from a more concentrated solution, we can use the following formula:

$$C_1 V_1 = C_2 V_2$$

In this particular case, the following values apply:

- $C_1 = 25\%$.
- $V_1 = $ Unknown.
- $C_2 = 7\%$.
- $V_2 = 35 \, mL$.

Therefore, entering the values into the equation, you get:

$$25 \times V_1 = 7 \times 35.$$

$$25 \times V_1 = 245.$$

$$V_1 = 245 \div 25.$$

$$V_1 = 9.8 \, mL.$$

Therefore, you will require 9.8 mL of a 25% solution of Drug G to make 35 mL of a 7% solution.

**QUESTION 6.11:** *Check the answer you obtained for Question 6.10 by working through the calculation as described in Example 6:11.*

**ANSWER:**    You stated that you require 9.8 mL of a 25% solution of Drug G to make 35 mL of a 7% solution.

A 25% solution will contain 25 g of Drug G in every 100 mL. Therefore, in 9.8 mL, there would be:

$$(25 \div 100) \times 9.8 = 2.45 \, g.$$

This amount of drug would be dissolved in 35 mL of solution to produce a solution of the following concentration:

$$(2.45 \div 35) \times 100 = 7\%.$$

---

**QUESTION 6.12:** *You are told that 360 mL of a 12% w/v solution of Drug H was used to make 1 L of a final solution. What is the concentration of this final solution?*

**ANSWER:**    We can use the following formula:

$$C_1 V_1 = C_2 V_2$$

In this particular case, the following values apply:

- $C_1 = 12\%$.
- $V_1 = 360 \, mL$.
- $C_2 = $ Unknown.
- $V_2 = 1 \, L \, (1000 \, mL)$.

Therefore, entering the values into the equation, you get:

$$12 \times 360 = C_2 \times 1000.$$
$$4320 = C_2 \times 1000.$$
$$C_2 = 4320 \div 1000.$$
$$C_2 = 4.32\%.$$

Therefore, you will produce a 4.32% solution by diluting 360 mL of a 12% solution of Drug H to 1 L.

---

**QUESTION 6.13:** *You are required to make 2.3 L of a 6.5% w/v solution of Drug I from a 16% solution. How much of the concentrated solution is required? Once calculated, check the answer by working through the calculation as described in Example 6:11.*

**ANSWER:**    We can use the following formula:

$$C_1 V_1 = C_2 V_2$$

In this particular case, the following values apply:

- $C_1 = 16\%$.
- $V_1 = $ Unknown.
- $C_2 = 6.5\%$.
- $V_2 = 2.3 \, L \, (2300 \, mL)$.

Therefore, entering the values into the equation, you get:

$16 \times V_1 = 6.5 \times 2300$.

$16 \times V_1 = 14\,950$.

$V_1 = 14\,950 \div 16$.

$V_1 = 934.375\,mL$.

Therefore, you will require 934.375 mL of a 16% solution of Drug I to make 2.3 L of a 6.5% solution.

To check, we said that you will require 934.375 mL of a 16% solution of Drug I to make 2.3 L of a 6.5% solution.

In 934.375 mL of a 16% solution, we would have:

16% is 16 g or 16 mL in 100 mL.

$(16 \div 100) \times 934.375 = 149.5\,g$ (or 149.5 mL).

149.5 g (or 149.5 mL) in 2.3 L (2300 mL) would produce:

$(149.5 \div 2300) \times 100 = 6.5\%$.

Therefore, 934.375 mL of a 16% solution does make 2.3 L of a 6.5% solution.

---

**QUESTION 6.14:** *You are asked to produce 350 g of a 4.6% cream using stock creams of 10% and 3%. How much of each stock cream will you require?*

**ANSWER:** As this question asks for a particular strength of a product to be made, from two other products, one of a higher and one of a lower strength, you need to use the alligation grid (Figure 6.1) to calculate the required proportions of each ingredient.

In this particular case, the following values are calculated:

- Proportion of higher strength product required = $4.6 - 3 = 1.6$.
- Proportion of lower strength product required = $10 - 4.6 = 5.4$.
- Therefore, the ratio of higher strength to lower strength is 1.6 to 5.4.

Then, to calculate the quantity of each ingredient, we need to work out the weight of each part. In total, we require 7 parts (1.6 + 5.4) and a total weight of 350 g.

Therefore, each part weighs $350 \div 7 = 50\,g$.

This means that the quantity of the two products to be mixed would be:

Quantity of higher strength product = $1.6 \times 50 = 80\,g$.

Quantity of lower strength product = $5.4 \times 50 = 270\,g$.

Therefore, you need to mix 80 g of 10% cream with 270 g of 3% cream to produce 350 g of 4.6% cream.

---

**QUESTION 6.15:** *Check the answer you obtained for Question 6.14 by working through the calculation as described in Example 6:13.*

**ANSWER:** In Question 6.14, we calculated that 80 g of 10% cream mixed with 270 g of 3% cream would produce 350 g of 4.6% cream.

To check this calculation, we need to calculate the amount of actual drug each cream would contribute to the final product, and then work out the resultant strength of the final product.

The higher strength product contains the active ingredient at 10% strength. This means that there are 10 g (or mL) of active ingredient per 100 g. If we are using 80 g of this product, there will be:

- $(10 \div 100) \times 80 = 8$ g (or mL).

The lower strength product contains the active ingredient at 3% strength. This means that there are 3 g (or mL) of active ingredient per 100 g. If we are using 270 g of this product, there will be:

- $(3 \div 100) \times 270 = 8.1$ g (or mL).

Therefore, in the total 350 g of product, there will be:

- $8 + 8.1 = 16.1$ g (or mL) of active ingredient.

This will produce a product of the following strength:

- $(16.1 \div 350) \times 100 = 4.6\%$.

As 4.6% was the desired strength, it means that the calculation in Question 6.14 is correct.

---

**QUESTION 6.16:** *You are asked to produce 75 g of a 13.5% cream using stock cream of 5.5% and the active ingredient. How much of the stock cream and the active ingredient (each to two decimal places) will you require?*

**ANSWER:**   As before, we can use the alligation grid (Figure 6.1) to calculate the required proportions of each ingredient.

In this particular case, the following values are calculated:

- Proportion of higher strength product required = $13.5 - 5.5 = 8$.
- Proportion of lower strength product required = $100 - 13.5 = 86.5$.
- Therefore, the ratio of higher strength to lower strength is 8 to 86.5.

Then, to calculate the quantity of each ingredient, we need to work out the weight of each part. In total, we require 94.5 parts (8 + 86.5) and a total weight of 75 g.

Therefore, each part weighs $75 \div 94.5 = 0.79$ g (to two decimal places).

This means that the quantity of the two products to be mixed would be:

Quantity of active ingredient = $8 \times (75 \div 94.5) = 6.35$ g (to two decimal places).

Quantity of lower strength product = $86.5 \times (75 \div 94.5) = 68.65$ g (to two decimal places).

Therefore, you need to mix 68.65 g of 5.5% cream with 6.35 g of active ingredient to produce 75 g of 13.5% cream.

---

**QUESTION 6.17:** *Check the answer you obtained for Question 6.16 by working through the calculation as described in Example 6:17.*

**ANSWER:**   In Question 6.16, we calculated that 68.65 g of 5.5% cream mixed with 6.35 g of active ingredient would produce 75 g of 13.5% cream.

To check this calculation, we need to calculate the amount of actual drug each ingredient would contribute to the final product, and then work out the resultant strength of the final product.

The higher strength product contains pure active ingredient (i.e. 100%). This means that there are 6.35 g of active ingredient being added to the lower strength cream.

The lower strength product contains the active ingredient at 5.5% strength. This means that there are 5.5 g of active ingredient per 100 g. If we are using 68.65 g of this product, there will be:

- $(5.5 \div 100) \times 68.65 = 3.78$ g (to two decimal places).

Therefore, in the total 75 g of product, there will be:

- $3.78 + 6.35 = 10.13$ g of active ingredient.

This will produce a product of the following strength:

- $(10.13 \div 75) \times 100 = 13.5\%$.

As 13.5% was the desired strength, it means that the calculation in Question 6.16 is correct.

---

**QUESTION 6.18:**

*Evie Jones has a skin complaint and the doctor has prescribed a cream at a strength of 3.5%. The only products available have percentages of 1% and 4.5%. The doctor has requested a supply of 120 g. How much of each cream needs to be mixed together to produce 120 g at the desired strength?*

**ANSWER:**

As this question asks for a particular strength of a product to be made, from two other products, one of a higher and one of a lower strength, you need to use the alligation grid (Figure 6.1) to calculate the required proportions of each ingredient.

In this particular case, the following values are calculated:

- Proportion of higher strength product required = $3.5 - 1 = 2.5$.
- Proportion of lower strength product required = $4.5 - 3.5 = 1$.
- Therefore, the ratio of higher strength to lower strength is 2.5 to 1.

Then, to calculate the quantity of each ingredient, we need to work out the weight of each part. In total, we require 3.5 parts $(1 + 2.5)$ and a total weight of 120 g.

Therefore, each part weighs $120 \div 3.5 = 34.29$ g (to two decimal places).

This means that the quantity of the two products to be mixed would be:

Quantity of higher strength product = $2.5 \times (120 \div 3.5) = 85.71$ g (to two decimal places).

Quantity of lower strength product = $1 \times (120 \div 3.5) = 34.29$ g.

Therefore, you need to mix 85.71 g of 4.5% cream with 34.29 g of 1% cream to produce 120 g of 3.5% cream.

To check this calculation, firstly check that the two quantities calculated add up to the desired total.

85.71 g + 34.29 g = 120 g.

Then we need to calculate the amount of actual drug each cream would contribute to the final product, and then work out the resultant strength of the final product.

The higher strength product contains the active ingredient at 4.5% strength. This means that there are 4.5 g (or mL) of active ingredient per 100 g. If we are using 85.71 g of this product, there will be:

- (4.5 ÷ 100) × 85.71 = 3.86 g (or mL) (to two decimal places).

The lower strength product contains the active ingredient at 1% strength. This means that there is 1 g (or mL) of active ingredient per 100 g. If we are using 34.29 g of this product, there will be:

- (1 ÷ 100) × 34.29 = 0.34 g (or mL) (to two decimal places).

Therefore, in the total 120 g of product, there will be:

- 3.86 + 0.34 = 4.2 g (or mL) of active ingredient.

This will produce a product of the following strength:

- (4.2 ÷ 120) × 100 = 3.5%.

As 3.5% was the desired strength, it means that the calculation above is correct.

**QUESTION 6.19:**

*Emma requires a solution every 6 hours to control her asthma. The dose of the drug is 5 mg/kg, four times a day. You are required to produce sufficient solution for 5 days' supply to allow each dose to be 10 mL using a 30% w/v stock solution. What quantity of stock solution is required?*

**ANSWER:**

Firstly, you need to calculate the dose based on Emma's weight. As Emma weighs 20.4 kg, the dose she requires is:

5 × 20.4 = 102 mg four times a day.

If the prescribed course is for 5 days, the total amount of drug required is:

102 × 4 × 5 = 2040 mg.

And the total volume to produce (based on a dosage volume of 10 mL) is:

10 × 4 × 5 = 200 mL.

If 2040 mg (2.04 g) is dissolved in 200 mL (assuming that the solubility of the active ingredient in the vehicle will allow this to happen), this would produce a solution with the following strength:

(2.04 ÷ 200) × 100 = 1.02%

Therefore, we now know that we need to produce 200 mL of a 1.02% solution from a 30% solution.

We can now use the following formula:

$C_1 V_1 = C_2 V_2$

In this particular case, the following values apply:

- $C_1 = 30\%$.
- $V_1 = $ Unknown.
- $C_2 = 1.02\%$.
- $V_2 = 200$ mL.

Therefore, entering the values into the equation, you get:

$30 \times V_1 = 1.02 \times 200$.

$30 \times V_1 = 204$.

$V_1 = 204 \div 30$.

$V_1 = 6.8$ mL.

Therefore, you will require 6.8 mL of a 30% solution to make 200 mL of a 1.02% solution.

To check, we said that you will require 6.8 mL of a 30% solution to make 200 mL of a 1.02% solution.

In 6.8 mL of a 30% solution, we would have:

30% is 30 g (or 30 mL) in 100 mL.

$(30 \div 100) \times 6.8 = 2.04$ g (or 2.04 mL).

2.04 g (or 2.04 mL) in 200 mL would produce:

$(2.04 \div 200) \times 100 = 1.02\%$

Therefore, 6.8 mL of a 30% solution does make 200 mL of a 1.02% solution.

If we administer 10 mL of this solution to Emma at each administration point, we would be giving her:

$1.02\% = 1.02$ g in every 100 mL.

Therefore, in 10 mL there would be: $(1.02 \div 100) \times 10 = 0.102$ g (102 mg).

As Emma weighs 20.4 kg, this is a dose of:

$102 \div 20.4 = 5$ mg/kg (as requested).

# Intravenous and associated medication routes

## 7.1 Chapter introduction

Following on from Chapter 6, where we discussed the calculations involved in the preparation of liquid and solid dosage forms for oral administration or topical application, this chapter will discuss the calculations involved in the preparation and administration of medication intended for administration intravenously or via associated routes (e.g. subcutaneously). This will include calculations designed to derive the appropriate administration rate for intravenous infusions, solution calculations based on medication administration rates, and the calculations involved in the conversion between oral and intravenous and associated dosages.

Up until this point, most of the calculations we have encountered relate to the administration of medication via the oral route. This is the most common route of administration for medication owing to the relative ease of administration when compared with other routes. As patients are able to self-administer medication via the oral route (or parents/carers are able to administer on behalf of a patient), this makes the oral route the primary choice in many medication regimens.

However, there are situations in which it may be preferable to administer medication via the intravenous route. It could be, for example, that because of the physicochemical properties of the drug other routes are not suitable (e.g. a drug which is easily degraded and so would not be suitable for oral administration) or where a rapid plasma level is required (e.g. for use within emergency medicine with unconscious patients). In these cases, it is necessary to be able to calculate infusion rates for medication.

## 7.2 Basic intravenous infusion rates

This section will discuss the calculations involved in the administration of medication via basic infusion rates; these are calculations where the infusion rate remains constant throughout the administration period. Section 7.3 will describe calculations where the administration rate changes at one or more points during the administration period.

This section is divided into three sub-sections:

- Section 7.2.1 will cover the calculations required to establish the amount of drug (or drug solution) needed to produce an infusion to deliver the intended dosage.
- Section 7.2.2 will discuss the steps involved in the calculation of infusion administration rates.
- Finally, section 7.2.3 will examine calculations looking at infusion volume.

## 7.2.1 Intravenous solution calculations

Basic infusion rates are normally expressed as an amount of drug to be administered over a set period of time. In Example 7:1, you are provided with both the dosage of medication the patient requires, and the administration rate (in mL/min), and you are asked to calculate the quantity of a drug required to make the infusion solution of a particular volume.

| | EXAMPLE 7:1 |
|---|---|
| Question: | You are asked to calculate the amount of Drug A required to make 500 mL of infusion where the administration rate is 5 mL/min and the dose is 100 micrograms/min. |
| Answer: | In this case, three pieces of information are available: the required volume of the final solution for infusion, the infusion rate (in volume per set time), and the dose (in quantity of drug per minute). From the latter two pieces of information, it is possible to calculate the strength of the solution.<br><br>If the administration rate is 5 mL/min and the dose is 100 micrograms/min, then the strength of the solution is 100 micrograms/5 mL.<br><br>Once we have calculated the strength of the solution, we can calculate the total quantity of Drug A for the required volume.<br><br>If there are 100 micrograms in every 5 mL, in 500 mL there are:<br><br>$(100 \div 5) \times 500 = 10\,000$ micrograms $\equiv 10$ mg.<br><br>Therefore, we require 10 mg of Drug A to make 500 mL of infusion where the administration rate is 5 mL/min and the dose is 100 micrograms/min. |

In Example 7:1 you calculated the quantity of a drug required to make a solution of a fixed volume. Although there are cases in which the infusion will be manufactured using the individual drug and a suitable vehicle, it is more common that a more concentrated solution of the drug (e.g. from a vial intended for an intravenous bolus dose) is added to a pre-prepared infusion solution (e.g. 0.9% sodium chloride or 5% dextrose). In these cases it is necessary to:

a) Calculate the quantity of the more concentrated solution required.

b) Remove the corresponding amount from the pre-prepared infusion solution before adding the concentrated solution.

This latter stage is required, firstly, to maintain the desired infusion volume (as unless the additional volume to be added is taken into consideration at the calculation stage, the final volume will be different, thus altering the concentration of the infusion solution), and, secondly, because the pre-prepared infusion bags are a fixed volume and may not have the space for the additional volume to be added. Example 7:2 demonstrates this additional calculation step.

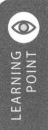

## Adding drug solutions to infusion bags

When adding concentrated drug solutions to infusion bags you need to remember to remove the corresponding volume before adding the drug, to maintain the desired final volume.

LEARNING POINT

| | **EXAMPLE 7:2** |
|---|---|
| **Question:** | You are asked to calculate the amount of a solution of Drug B required to make 250 mL of infusion where the administration rate is 2 mL/min and the dose is 500 micrograms/min. The solution of Drug B is 50 mg/10 mL. |
| **Answer:** | Three pieces of information are available: the required volume of the final solution for infusion, the infusion rate (in volume per set time) and the dose (in quantity of drug per minute). In addition, the strength of the concentrated solution to be used is also provided. From the infusion rate and dose, it is possible to calculate the strength of the solution. |

If the administration rate is 2 mL/min and the dose is 500 micrograms/min, then the strength of the solution is 500 micrograms/2 mL.

Once we have calculated the strength of the solution, we can calculate the total quantity of Drug B for the required volume.

If there are 500 micrograms in every 2 mL, in 250 mL there are:

$(500 \div 2) \times 250 = 62\,500$ micrograms $\equiv 62.5$ mg.

Therefore, we require 62.5 mg of Drug B to make 250 mL of infusion where the administration rate is 2 mL/min and the dose is 500 micrograms/min.

However, unlike Example 7:1, in this case the drug is coming from a more concentrated solution. Therefore, we need to calculate the volume of this solution required to provide the correct quantity of Drug B.

If the solution contains 50 mg/10 mL, for 62.5 mg, we require:

$(10 \div 50) \times 62.5 = 12.5$ mL.

Therefore, we need to add 12.5 mL of the 50 mg/10 mL solution of Drug B to a 250 mL infusion bag (remembering to remove a corresponding 12.5 mL first to maintain the final volume at 250 mL) to make 250 mL of infusion where the administration rate is 2 mL/min and the dose is 500 micrograms/min.

In Example 7:1 and Example 7:2, we were required to calculate the strength of a fixed volume of an infusion based on a given dosage and administration rate, and to use this to calculate the quantity of drug (or drug solution) required to make the final infusion solution. Example 7:3 contains a similar question but, in this case, you are asked to calculate the final volume of a fixed concentration required based on an administration time. Other questions examining infusion volume calculations can be found in section 7.2.3.

| | EXAMPLE 7:3 |
|---|---|
| **Question:** | You are asked to calculate the volume of a solution of Drug C, and the quantity of drug required, where the administration rate is 0.6 mL/min and the dose is 500 micrograms/min. The infusion is required for 5 hours. |
| **Answer:** | In this example, three pieces of information are available: the total administration time, the infusion rate (in volume per set time), and the dose (in quantity of drug per minute). From the latter two pieces of information, it is possible to calculate the strength of the solution.<br><br>If the administration rate is 0.6 mL/min and the dose is 500 micrograms/min, then the strength of the solution is 500 micrograms/0.6 mL.<br><br>Once we have calculated the strength of the solution, we can calculate the total volume required based on the administration rate.<br><br>If the administration rate is 0.6 mL/min and the infusion is required for 5 hours, the total volume required is:<br><br>$(0.6 \times 60) \times 5 = 180$ mL.<br><br>Finally, we are able to calculate the quantity of Drug C required:<br><br>If there are 500 micrograms in every 0.6 mL, in 180 mL there are:<br><br>$(500 \div 0.6) \times 180 = 150\,000$ micrograms $\equiv 150$ mg.<br><br>Therefore, we require 150 mg of Drug C, made up to a 180 mL infusion, for a 5-hour infusion where the administration rate is 0.6 mL/min and the dose is 500 micrograms/min. |

## 7.2.2 Infusion rate calculations

In section 7.2.1 we had to calculate the amount of medication (either actual drug or amount of drug solution) to be added to make a solution of a fixed volume based on previously known dosage and infusion rate. Although the preparation of individual solutions for infusion is undertaken, and it is therefore important to understand the calculations involved, it is also common to have to calculate the infusion rate required for infusion of a fixed concentration to provide a particular dose. Firstly, see Example 7:4 where we have to calculate the infusion rate required for the administration of a readily available solution.

| | EXAMPLE 7:4 |
|---|---|
| **Question:** | You are asked to calculate the infusion rate, in mL/hour, for a 2 L solution of Drug D at a concentration of 75 mg/200 mL and a required dosage of 250 micrograms/min. |

**Answer:**   If the dosage is 250 micrograms/min, we need to convert this to volume per hour first as the final administration rate is required in mL/hour.

$$250 \text{ micrograms/min} = 250 \times 60 = 15\,000 \text{ micrograms/hour.}$$

$$15\,000 \text{ micrograms/hour} \equiv 15 \text{ mg/hour.}$$

Once we have the administration rate in quantity of drug per hour, we can convert this to the volume of drug to be administered per hour.

The administration rate is 15 mg/hour and the solution has a concentration of 75 mg/200 mL. Therefore, each hour we require:

$$(200 \div 75) \times 15 = 40 \text{ mL.}$$

Therefore, the infusion rate is 40 mL/hour.

As with questions in previous chapters, it is useful to develop a self-checking technique for pharmaceutical calculations where you take the answer you have calculated and work back through the question to check. Example 7:5 does this for the answer obtained in Example 7:4.

| EXAMPLE 7:5 | |
|---|---|
| **Question:** | In Example 7:4 we stated that setting a 75 mg/200 mL solution at an infusion rate of 40 mL/hour would provide a dosage of 250 micrograms/minute. |
| **Answer:** | Firstly, we need to calculate how much drug is administered per hour and then convert this to an administration rate per minute. |
| | If there are 75 mg in every 200 mL of the infusion solution, in 40 mL, there would be: |
| | $(75 \div 200) \times 40 = 15$ mg of drug. |
| | This provides us with the amount of drug being administered per hour. Then this can be converted to an administration rate per minute. |
| | $15 \div 60 = 0.25$ mg/min or 250 micrograms/min. |
| | Therefore, a 75 mg/200 mL solution at an infusion rate of 40 mL/hour would provide a dosage of 250 micrograms/min. |

The same technique can be used to check the answers from section 7.2.1. Example 7:6 demonstrates how you can check the answer obtained from Example 7:1.

| EXAMPLE 7:6 | |
|---|---|
| **Question:** | In Example 7:1 we stated that we require 10 mg of Drug A to make 500 mL of infusion where the administration rate is 5 mL/min and the dose is 100 micrograms/min. |
| **Answer:** | There are two ways to check this, firstly to work out the amount of drug administered per minute. If we produce a solution with a concentration of 10 mg/500 mL and administer at a rate of 5 mL/min, the amount of drug administered per minute would be: |

$(10 \div 500) \times 5 = 0.1$ mg/minute $\equiv 100$ micrograms/min.

Alternatively, we can calculate the administration rate from the concentration of the solution and the dose. If we produce a solution with a concentration of 10 mg/500 mL and we want a dose of 100 micrograms/min, we firstly need to convert the concentration from milligrams to micrograms:

10 mg/500 mL $\equiv$ 10 000 micrograms/500 mL.

Then we can work out the quantity of this solution required, per minute, to give the required dose of 100 micrograms/min:

$(500 \div 10\,000) \times 100 = 5$ mL/min.

Therefore, 10 mg of Drug A will make 500 mL of infusion where the administration rate is 5 mL/min and the dose is 100 micrograms/min.

The other main types of basic infusion rate calculations are ones in which the dosage is linked to the weight of the patient. Take Example 7:7, which is similar to Example 7:1 but where the dosage is related to the weight of the patient.

| EXAMPLE 7:7 | |
|---|---|
| **Question:** | You are asked to calculate the amount of Drug E required to make 500 mL of infusion where the administration rate is 5 mL/min and the dose is 25 micrograms/kg/min. The patient weighs 60 kg. |
| **Answer:** | Three pieces of information are available: the required volume of the final solution for infusion, the infusion rate (in volume per set time), and the dose (in quantity of drug per kilogram of patient per minute). From the latter two pieces of information, it is possible to calculate the strength of the solution once the dosage has been converted from weight of drug per kilogram of patient per minute to the total weight of drug to be administered per minute. |
| | Firstly, convert the dosage using the patient's weight: |
| | If the dosage is 25 micrograms/kg/min and the patient weighs 60 kg, the dose is: |
| | $25 \times 60 = 1500$ micrograms/min $\equiv 1.5$ mg/min. |
| | If the administration rate is 5 mL/min and the dose is 1.5 mg/min, then the strength of the solution is 1.5 mg/5 mL. |
| | Once we have calculated the strength of the solution, we can calculate the total quantity of Drug E for the required volume. |
| | If there are 1.5 mg in every 5 mL, in 500 mL there are: |
| | $(1.5 \div 5) \times 500 = 150$ mg. |
| | Therefore, we require 150 mg of Drug E to make 500 mL of infusion where the administration rate is 5 mL/min and the dose is 25 micrograms/kg/min for a 60 kg patient. |

As with the previous calculations within this section, it is worth checking the answer by working through the calculation.

| | EXAMPLE 7:8 |
|---|---|
| **Question:** | In Example 7:7 we stated that we would require 150 mg of Drug E to make 500 mL of infusion where the administration rate is 5 mL/min and the dose is 25 micrograms/kg/min for a 60 kg patient. |
| **Answer:** | 150 mg of Drug E in 500 mL would make:<br><br>$\qquad 150 \div 500 = 0.3$ mg/mL $= 300$ micrograms/mL.<br><br>Then we can check the answer by either calculating the amount of drug to be administered per minute or the administration rate, in a similar way to Example 7:6. First, calculate the amount of drug to be administered per minute.<br><br>$\qquad$ If the solution contains 150 mg of Drug E in every 500 mL, in 5 mL (the amount administered per minute) there would be:<br><br>$\qquad (150 \div 500) \times 5 = 1.5$ mg/min.<br><br>To convert this to the original dose in micrograms/kg/min, we have to divide by the patient's weight. In this example, the patient weighs 60 kg.<br><br>$\qquad (1.5 \div 60) = 0.025$ mg/kg/min $\equiv 25$ micrograms/kg/min.<br><br>Alternatively, calculate the administration rate. If the dosage is 25 micrograms/kg/min and the patient weighs 60 kg, the dosage per minute is:<br><br>$\qquad 25 \times 60 = 1500$ micrograms/min.<br><br>1500 micrograms/minute would require an infusion rate (based on a solution concentration of 300 micrograms/mL) of:<br><br>$\qquad (1500 \div 300) = 5$ mL/min.<br><br>Therefore, 150 mg of Drug E is required for a 500 mL infusion where the administration rate is 5 mL/min and the dose is 25 micrograms/kg/min for a 60 kg patient. |

### 7.2.3 Infusion volume calculations

Finally, in this section we can examine calculations looking at the quantity of a solution required for a particular length of an infusion. For example, let's examine a situation where we are aware of the concentration of the infusion to be given and the infusion rate and we need to calculate the volume to be infused (see Example 7:9).

| | EXAMPLE 7:9 |
|---|---|
| **Question:** | Calculate the volume of solution required for an infusion of Drug F, at a concentration of 30 mg/25 mL, where you are asked to infuse a total of 900 mg. |
| **Answer:** | If a total of 900 mg is to be infused, and the concentration of the desired solution is 30 mg/25 mL, the total volume required is:<br><br>$\qquad (25 \div 30) \times 900 = 750$ mL.<br><br>Therefore, we will require a total of 750 mL of a 30 mg/25 mL solution of Drug F to infuse a total of 900 mg. |

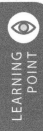

**Overage**

In practice, depending on the administration method employed, it is sometimes the case that an overage will be factored into the calculation to allow for the inability to infuse the entirety of the infusion solution. In this example, no overage is mentioned in the question and so it is not necessary to calculate an overage.

LEARNING POINT

An extension of the question in Example 7:9 would then ask you to calculate an infusion rate for the infusion to provide a particular dose; see Example 7:10.

| | **EXAMPLE 7:10** |
|---|---|
| **Question:** | At what rate would the infusion of Drug F from Example 7:9 need to be delivered to provide a dose of 6 mg/min? How long would the infusion last? |
| **Answer:** | Firstly, calculate the infusion rate. If 6 mg/min is required, we need to know the volume of solution that contains 6 mg. As the solution is 30 mg/25 mL, this would be: |
| | $(25 \div 30) \times 6 = 5$ mL/min. |
| | Next, we need to calculate how long the infusion will last. From the last calculation, we worked out that 5 mL of infusion would be administered every minute. Therefore, for 750 mL it would take: |
| | $(750 \div 5) = 150$ minutes or 2.5 hours. |
| | Therefore, the infusion of Drug F from Example 7:9 would need to be delivered at 5 mL/min to provide a dose of 6 mg/min. The infusion would last a total of 2.5 hours. |

## 7.3 Variable intravenous infusion rates

The examples covered in section 7.2 relate to the administration of medication via infusion where the rate is constant during the administration period. Other types of calculation will be used when there is a change to the administration rate, see Example 7:11.

| | **EXAMPLE 7:11** |
|---|---|
| **Question:** | An infusion of Drug G is to be delivered at a dose of 60 mg/kg/hour for 5 hours. After this time, the dose is reduced to 30 mg/kg/hour. How long would a 200 mL infusion bag at a concentration of 150 mg/0.5 mL last if the patient weighs 75 kg? |
| **Answer:** | To tackle this calculation we first need to work out how much drug will be required for the first 5 hours of infusion. If the dose is 60 mg/kg/hour and the patient weighs 75 kg, the amount of drug infused would be: |

$$60 \times 75 \times 5 = 22\,500 \text{ mg } (22.5 \text{ g}).$$

Then we need to calculate the volume of infusion that this administration period would require. If there are 150 mg/0.5 mL, for 22 500 mg, we would infuse:

$$(0.5 \div 150) \times 22\,500 = 75 \text{ mL}.$$

To work out how long the bag will last, we need to calculate the amount of time it will take to use the remainder of the bag after the infusion is reduced to an infusion rate of 30 mg/kg/hour. If the original bag was 200 mL and after 5 hours we have infused 75 mL, the remaining volume will be:

$$200 - 75 = 125 \text{ mL}.$$

If there are 125 mL remaining and the bag has a concentration of 150 mg/0.5 mL, the amount of Drug G remaining is:

$$(150 \div 0.5) \times 125 = 37\,500 \text{ mg } (37.5 \text{ g}).$$

At a (revised) administration rate of 30 mg/kg/hour and a patient weight of 75 kg, the revised rate per hour is:

$$30 \times 75 = 2250 \text{ mg/hour}.$$

Therefore, to use the remainder of Drug G (37 500 mg) it will take:

$$37\,500 \div 2250 = 16.67 \text{ hours (to two decimal places)} \equiv 16 \text{ hours } 40 \text{ minutes}.$$

Therefore, in total, it will last:

$$5 + 16.67 = 21.67 \text{ hours (to two decimal places) (21 hours, 40 minutes)}.$$

Example 7:12, provides a similar calculation question to Example 7:11 but in this example, the question asks how long it will take *for the remainder* of the infusion to be delivered (as opposed to the entire infusion as detailed within Example 7:11).

| EXAMPLE 7:12 | |
|---|---|
| **Question:** | An infusion of Drug H is to be delivered at a dose of 5 mg/kg/hour for 2.5 hours. After this time, the dose is increased to 7.5 mg/kg/hour. After the change of administration rate, how long would it take for the remainder of a 750 mL infusion bag at a concentration of 20 mg/mL to be administered if the patient weighs 80 kg? |
| **Answer:** | To tackle this calculation we first need to work out how much drug will be required for the first 2.5 hours of infusion. If the dose is 5 mg/kg/hour and the patient weighs 80 kg, the amount of drug infused would be: $$5 \times 80 \times 2.5 = 1000 \text{ mg } (1 \text{ g}).$$ Then we need to calculate the volume of infusion that this administration period would require. If there are 20 mg/mL, for 1000 mg, we would infuse: $$(1 \div 20) \times 1000 = 50 \text{ mL}.$$ |

To work out how long the remainder of the bag will last, we need to calculate the amount of time it will take to use the remainder of the bag after the infusion is increased to an infusion rate of 7.5 mg/kg/hour. If the original bag was 750 mL and after 2.5 hours we have infused 50 mL, the remaining volume will be:

750 − 50 = 700 mL.

If there are 700 mL remaining and the bag has a concentration of 20 mg/mL, the amount of Drug H remaining is:

$(20 \div 1) \times 700 = 14\,000$ mg (14 g).

At a (revised) administration rate of 7.5 mg/kg/hour and a patient weight of 80 kg, the revised rate per hour is:

$7.5 \times 80 = 600$ mg/hour.

Therefore, to use the remainder of Drug H (14 000 mg) it will take:

$14\,000 \div 600 = 23.33$ hours (to two decimal places) ≡ 23 hours 20 minutes.

Therefore, after the end of the first administration period it will take a further 23 hours and 20 minutes to administer the remainder of the infusion.

---

### Calculations involving a change in administration rate

In Example 7:11 and Example 7:12 we explored calculations involving a similar change in administration rate but where different answers are requested. In Example 7:11, you were asked to calculate the time taken to infuse the entire infusion (i.e. the combined total of the two administration periods). For Example 7:12 you were asked to calculate and provide the time taken for the remainder of the infusion after the administration rate was changed. When tackling questions of this type, ensure that you read the question fully and provide the answer to the actual question.

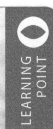

LEARNING POINT

---

## 7.4 Converting oral administration rates to other routes

One specific set of calculations relating to administration rates is the conversion of oral therapy to intravenous therapy for the treatment of pain. Although each individual's therapy should be monitored and titrated as appropriate following a switch, the *British National Formulary* provides guidance on approximate conversion values (see *Prescribing in palliative care* at the beginning of the book).

| | EXAMPLE 7:13 |
|---|---|
| Question: | A patient currently takes 20 mg of oral morphine twice a day (as sustained-release tablets). His doctor wants to change this to an intramuscular administration of diamorphine. What is the total daily dose of intramuscular diamorphine required? |

| **Answer:** | To convert oral morphine to intramuscular diamorphine, you need to consult the equivalent dosage table in the *British National Formulary* (see *Prescribing in palliative care*). This states that the equivalent dose of intramuscular diamorphine is approximately one-third the oral dose of morphine. Therefore, a twice-daily dose of 20 mg oral morphine is equivalent to: |
| --- | --- |

$$(20 \times 2) \div 3 = 13.33 \text{ mg (to two decimal places)}.$$

Therefore, the total daily dose of intramuscular diamorphine required is 13.33 mg (to two decimal places).

As detailed within *Prescribing in palliative care* in the *British National Formulary*, conversion of doses from oral to intramuscular administration for morphine can be calculated by working out half the oral dose, or for modified-release preparations, half the total daily oral dose, divided into six portions for 4-hourly administration.

**LEARNING POINT**

### Calculations involving a change in administration route

It is not uncommon for pharmacists or pharmacy technicians to be asked to convert medication dosages from one administration route to another. This is particularly the case for patients on analgesia where an oral dose may be converted to an intramuscular or intravenous dose as the disease state progresses. For these calculations it is important to consult appropriate reference sources for conversion details (e.g. the *British National Formulary*) and in practice, monitor the patient and titrate the dose via the new administration route as appropriate.

| | **EXAMPLE 7:14** |
| --- | --- |
| **Question:** | A patient currently takes 30 mg of oral morphine twice a day (as sustained-release tablets). Her doctor wants to change this to intramuscular administration. What is the dose of intramuscular morphine required? |
| **Answer:** | To convert oral morphine to intramuscular morphine, you need to halve the total daily dose and then divide into six (4-hourly) portions (see *Prescribing in palliative care* within the *British National Formulary*). Therefore, a twice-daily dose of 30 mg oral morphine is equivalent to a daily intramuscular dose of: |

$$(30 \times 2) \div 2 = 30 \text{ mg}.$$

This would produce a 4-hourly dose of:

$$30 \div 6 = 5 \text{ mg}.$$

Therefore, the intramuscular morphine should be administered at a dose of 5 mg every 4 hours.

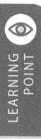

## 4-hourly and 6-hourly dosages

You need to be careful with 4-hourly and 6-hourly dosages. As there are 24 hours in a day, a 6-hourly dose will be administered four times a day and a 4-hourly dose six times a day. As these different dosages differ by the transposition of 'four' and 'six', it can be easy to make a mistake with dosages involving 4-hourly and 6-hourly dosages.

# 7.5 Infusion administration methods

The examples in sections 7.2, 7.3, and 7.4 do not specify the infusion administration method used. However, variations of these calculations may require an additional step or steps to be added to the calculation to accommodate the chosen administration methodology. In essence, there are two main methods for the infusion of medication: via an electronic syringe driver (see section 7.5.1) or via a drip (see section 7.5.2).

## 7.5.1 Calculations involving electronic syringe drivers

Although the basics of electronic syringe driver calculations have been covered in the preceding sections within this chapter, you may also be asked to calculate administration rates based on the individual syringe attached to the electronic syringe driver. Essentially, an electronic syringe driver is a machine that depresses the plunger on a syringe of medication at a set speed. Figure 7.1 provides an example of an electronic syringe driver.

As you can see from Figure 7.1, the syringe of medication is placed on the syringe driver and the machine's arm attached to the end of the plunger. The machine will then be programmed to depress the plunger at a fixed speed. For some systems, the details of the medication strength and volume can be entered into the machine along with the required dose, and the rate at which the plunger is depressed will be calculated.

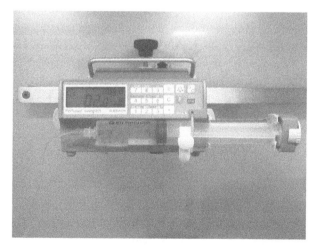

**Figure 7.1** An electronic syringe driver. This file is licensed under the Creative Commons Attribution-Share Alike 3.0 Germany license. Copyright: Philipp Lensing.

Alternatively, it may be necessary to calculate the administration rate manually. In both cases, it is necessary to be familiar with these types of calculation to enable administration rates to be checked manually.

| | **EXAMPLE 7:15** |
|---|---|
| **Question:** | A patient requires a dose of 30 mg/hour of Drug I. The solution in the syringe is 75 mg/5 mL and the syringe contains 50 mL and is 10 cm long. At what administration rate, in mm/hour, is the machine required to be set? |
| **Answer:** | This calculation is similar to ones encountered earlier in this chapter only the administration rate is required in length per hour rather than volume per hour. Firstly, calculate the volume of drug required per hour. If the dose is 30 mg/hour and the solution is at a concentration of 75 mg/5 mL, the volume of drug required per hour is: $$(5 \div 75) \times 30 = 2 \text{ mL/hour.}$$ Next, work out the length of the syringe which contains this volume. If we consider that the syringe is a fixed cylinder of 50 mL volume and 10 cm length, each cm of length is equivalent to: $$50 \div 10 = 5 \text{ mL.}$$ Therefore, the required 2 mL will be the equivalent of: $$2 \div 5 = 0.4 \text{ cm} \equiv 4 \text{ mm.}$$ This means that for a dose of 30 mg/hour of Drug I, a 50 mL syringe of 10 cm length containing a solution of 75 mg/5 mL needs to be set at an administration rate of 4 mm/hour. |

### 7.5.2 Calculations involving drips

The other infusion methodology involves the administration of an infusion via a drip. In this case, the medication for infusion is held on a pole about the height of the patient and gravity is used to draw the medication from the bag. To regulate the flow, the medication exits the bag through an aperture that can be altered to allow a certain number of drops per unit of time. By knowing the volume of each drop, it is possible to calculate the infusion rate. Figure 7.2 shows two infusion bags and giving sets arranged for administration.

| | **EXAMPLE 7:16** |
|---|---|
| **Question:** | A patient requires a dose of 12.5 mg/hour of Drug J. The solution in the infusion bag is 1.5 mg/15 mL and the bag contains 500 mL. The bag is set up on a giving set with a drop volume of 0.1 mL. At what drop rate (drops per minute) does the giving set need to be set? |
| **Answer:** | This calculation is similar to ones encountered earlier in this chapter only the administration rate is required in drops per minute rather than volume per time period. Firstly, calculate the volume of drug required per minute. If the dose is 12.5 mg/hour and the solution is at a concentration of 1.5 mg/15 mL, the volume of drug required per hour is: |

$(12.5 \div 1.5) \times 15 = 125$ mL/hour.

Next, convert this to a volume per minute.

$125 \div 60 = 2.08$ mL/min (to two decimal places).

Then convert this volume to drops based on each drop having a volume of 0.1 mL.

$(125 \div 60) \div 0.1 = 20.83$ drops/min (to two decimal places). As in other similar calculations, to reduce any error caused by decimal places the fraction was left as '$125 \div 60$' rather than '2.08' in the last calculation.

Therefore, to the nearest drop, we need to set the giving set to 21 drops/min to provide a dose of 12.5 mg/hour of Drug J if the solution in the infusion bag is 1.5 mg/15 mL.

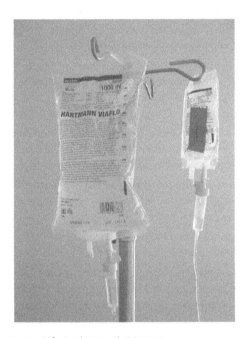

**Figure 7.2** A drip showing two infusion bags and giving sets.

# 7.6 Self-assessment questions

## 7.6.1 Basic self-assessment questions

This section contains a number of basic self-assessment questions for you to undertake to ensure that you have an understanding of the material in this chapter. It is recommended that you undertake all of these calculations **without a calculator** and then check your answers with the answers in section 7.8.

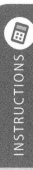

INSTRUCTIONS

**The use of calculators for the self-assessment questions in this chapter**

It is recommended that you undertake the following calculations without the use of a calculator.

All of the self-assessment questions within this section can be undertaken using a pen and paper.

**QUESTION 7.1:**   *You are asked to calculate the amount of Drug A required to make 750 mL of infusion where the administration rate is 10 mL/min and the dose is 250 micrograms/min.*

**QUESTION 7.2:**   *Check the answer you obtained for Question 7.1 by working through the calculation as described in Example 7:6.*

**QUESTION 7.3:**   *You are asked to calculate the amount of a solution of Drug B required to make 500 mL of infusion where the administration rate is 2.5 mL/min and the dose is 150 micrograms/min. The solution of Drug B is 75 mg/5 mL.*

**QUESTION 7.4:**   *You are asked to calculate the volume of a solution of Drug C and the quantity of drug required where the administration rate is 0.8 mL/min and the dose is 160 micrograms/min. The infusion is required for 6 hours.*

**QUESTION 7.5:**   *You are asked to calculate the infusion rate, in mL/hour for a 5 L solution of Drug D at a concentration of 12.5 mg/20 mL and a required dosage of 300 micrograms/min.*

**QUESTION 7.6:**   *Check the answer you obtained for Question 7.5 by working through the calculation as described in Example 7:5.*

**QUESTION 7.7:**   *You are asked to calculate the amount of Drug E required to make 2.3 L of infusion where the administration rate is 5 mL/min and the dose is 60 micrograms/kg/min. The patient weighs 80 kg.*

**QUESTION 7.8:**   *Check the answer you obtained for Question 7.7 by working through the calculation as described in Example 7:8.*

**QUESTION 7.9:**   *Calculate the volume of solution required (to two decimal places) for an infusion of Drug F, at a concentration of 65 mg/30 mL, where you are asked to infuse a total of 500 mg.*

**QUESTION 7.10:**   *At what rate (to two decimal places) would the infusion of Drug F from Question 7.9 need to be delivered to provide a dose of 7.5 mg/min? How long would the infusion last (to the nearest minute)?*

**QUESTION 7.11:**   *An infusion of Drug G is to be delivered at a dose of 30 mg/kg/hour for 10 hours. After this time, the dose is reduced to 5 mg/kg/hour. How long would a 500 mL infusion bag at a concentration of 250 mg/1.5 mL last if the patient weighs 78 kg?*

**QUESTION 7.12:**   *An infusion of Drug H is to be delivered at a dose of 35 mg/kg/hour for 3 hours. After this time, the dose is decreased to 20 mg/kg/hour. After the change of administration rate, how long (to the nearest minute) would it take for the remainder of a 1 L infusion bag at a concentration of 15 mg/mL to be administered if the patient weighs 65 kg?*

**QUESTION 7.13:**   *A patient currently takes 35 mg of oral morphine twice a day (as sustained-release tablets). His doctor wants to change this to an intramuscular administration of diamorphine. What is the total daily dose of intramuscular diamorphine required? See* Prescribing in palliative care *within the current edition of the* British National Formulary *(and Example 7:13).*

**QUESTION 7.14:**   *A patient currently takes 45 mg of oral morphine twice a day (as sustained-release tablets). Her doctor wants to change this to intramuscular administration. What is the dose of intramuscular morphine required? Note: see* Prescribing in palliative care *within the current edition of the* British National Formulary *(and Example 7:14).*

**QUESTION 7.15:**   *A patient requires a dose of 45 mg/hour of Drug I. The solution in the syringe is 25 mg/5 mL and the syringe contains 50 mL and is 10 cm long. At what administration rate, in mm/hour, is the machine required to be set?*

**QUESTION 7.16:**   *A patient requires a dose of 270 mg/hour of Drug J. The solution in the infusion bag is 75 mg/10 mL and the bag contains 250 mL. The bag is set up on a giving set with a drop volume of 0.1 mL. At what drop rate (drops per minute) does the giving set need to be set?*

### 7.6.2 Running case studies

**QUESTION 7.17:**

*Roger has been admitted to hospital to enable his pain to be controlled. He has been taking one 30 mg sustained-release morphine tablet every 12 hours but his doctor wants to change him onto a subcutaneous dosage of diamorphine. With reference to the current* British National Formulary, *advise the doctor what the daily dose of subcutaneous diamorphine would be.*

**QUESTION 7.18:**

*Geoff has been admitted to hospital and has been prescribed an antibiotic at 12 mg/kg/hour. The solution in the syringe is 250 mg/5 mL and the syringe contains 50 mL and is 10 cm long. At what administration rate, in mm/hour, is the machine required to be set?*

# 7.7 Summary

This chapter has provided examples and self-assessment questions surrounding the topic of intravenous and associated medication routes. Calculations around simple infusion rates have been covered, along with infusion volume calculations and those calculations relating to variable intravenous infusion rates. In addition, the important role the pharmacist and pharmacy technician can play in the calculations required in the transfer of a patient's medication from an oral to an alternative route of administration has been covered. Calculations involving modern electronic syringe drivers have been described, in addition to those relating to the more traditional drip method of administration.

## 7.8 Answers to self-assessment questions

This section contains the worked answers for the self-assessment questions within section 7.6.

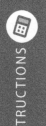

### The use of calculators for the self-assessment questions in this chapter

It is recommended that you undertake the following calculations without the use of a calculator.

All of the self-assessment questions within this section can be undertaken using a pen and paper.

**INSTRUCTIONS**

---

**QUESTION 7.1:**    *You are asked to calculate the amount of Drug A required to make 750 mL of infusion where the administration rate is 10 mL/min and the dose is 250 micrograms/min.*

**ANSWER:**    From the infusion rate (in volume per set time) and the dose (in weight of drug per minute), it is possible to calculate the strength of the solution.

If the administration rate is 10 mL/min and the dose is 250 micrograms/min, then the strength of the solution is 250 micrograms/10 mL.

Once we have calculated the strength of the solution, we can calculate the total quantity of Drug A for the required volume.

If there are 250 micrograms in every 10 mL, in 750 mL there are:

$(250 \div 10) \times 750 = 18\,750$ micrograms $\equiv 18.75$ mg.

Therefore, we require 18.75 mg of Drug A to make 750 mL of infusion where the administration rate is 10 mL/min and the dose is 250 micrograms/min.

---

**QUESTION 7.2:**    *Check the answer you obtained for Question 7.1 by working through the calculation as described in Example 7:6.*

**ANSWER:**    In the answer to Question 7.1 we stated that we require 18.75 mg of Drug A to make 750 mL of infusion where the administration rate is 10 mL/min and the dose is 250 micrograms/min.

There are two ways to check this, firstly to work out the amount of drug administered per minute. If we produce a solution with a concentration of 18.75 mg/750 mL and administer it at a rate of 10 mL/min, the amount of drug administered per minute would be:

$$(18.75 \div 750) \times 10 = 0.25 \text{ mg/min} \equiv 250 \text{ micrograms/min}.$$

Alternatively, we can calculate the administration rate from the concentration of the solution and the dose. If we produce a solution with a concentration of 18.75 mg/750 mL and we want a dose of 250 micrograms/min, we firstly need to convert the concentration from milligrams to micrograms:

$$18.75 \text{ mg/750 mL} \equiv 18\,750 \text{ micrograms/750 mL}.$$

Then we can work out the quantity of this solution required, per minute, to give the required dose of 250 micrograms/min:

$$(750 \div 18\,750) \times 250 = 10 \text{ mL/min}.$$

Therefore, 18.75 mg of Drug A will make 750 mL of infusion where the administration rate is 10 mL/min and the dose is 250 micrograms/min.

---

**QUESTION 7.3:** *You are asked to calculate the amount of a solution of Drug B required to make 500 mL of infusion where the administration rate is 2.5 mL/min and the dose is 150 micrograms/min. The solution of Drug B is 75 mg/5 mL.*

**ANSWER:** If the administration rate is 2.5 mL/min and the dose is 150 micrograms/min, then the strength of the solution is 150 micrograms/2.5 mL.

Once we have calculated the strength of the solution, we can calculate the total quantity of Drug B for the required volume.

If there are 150 micrograms in every 2.5 mL, in 500 mL there are:

$$(150 \div 2.5) \times 500 = 30\,000 \text{ micrograms} \equiv 30 \text{ mg}.$$

Therefore, we require 30 mg of Drug B to make 500 mL of infusion where the administration rate is 2.5 mL/min and the dose is 150 micrograms/min.

Next, we need to calculate the volume of this solution required to provide the correct quantity of Drug B.

If the solution contains 75 mg/5 mL, for 30 mg, we require:

$$(5 \div 75) \times 30 = 2 \text{ mL}.$$

Therefore, we need to add 2 mL of the 75 mg/5 mL to a 500 mL infusion bag (remembering to remove a corresponding 2 mL first to maintain the final volume at 500 mL) to make 500 mL of infusion, where the administration rate is 2.5 mL/min and the dose is 150 micrograms/min.

---

**QUESTION 7.4:** *You are asked to calculate the volume of a solution of Drug C and the quantity of drug required where the administration rate is 0.8 mL/min and the dose is 160 micrograms/min. The infusion is required for 6 hours.*

**ANSWER:** If the administration rate is 0.8 mL/min and the dose is 160 micrograms/min, then the strength of the solution is 160 micrograms/0.8 mL.

Once we have calculated the strength of the solution, we can calculate the total volume required based on the administration rate.

If the administration rate is 0.8 mL/min and the infusion is required for 6 hours, the total volume required is:

$(0.8 \times 60) \times 6 = 288$ mL.

Finally, we are able to calculate the quantity of Drug C required:

If there are 160 micrograms in every 0.8 mL, in 288 mL there are:

$(160 \div 0.8) \times 288 = 57\,600$ micrograms $\equiv 57.6$ mg.

Therefore, we require 57.6 mg of Drug C, made up to a 288 mL infusion for a 6-hour infusion where the administration rate is 0.8 mL/min and the dose is 160 micrograms/min.

**QUESTION 7.5:** *You are asked to calculate the infusion rate, in mL/hour for a 5 L solution of Drug D at a concentration of 12.5 mg/20 mL and a required dosage of 300 micrograms/min.*

**ANSWER:** If the dosage is 300 micrograms/min, we need to convert this to volume per hour first as the final administration rate is required in mL/hour.

300 micrograms/min = $300 \times 60 = 18\,000$ micrograms/hour.

18 000 micrograms/hour $\equiv 18$ mg/hour.

Once we have the administration rate in quantity of drug per hour, we can convert this to the volume of drug to be administered per hour.

The administration rate is 18 mg/hour and the solution has a concentration of 12.5 mg/20 mL. Therefore, each hour we require:

$(20 \div 12.5) \times 18 = 28.8$ mL.

Therefore, the infusion rate is 28.8 mL/hour.

**QUESTION 7.6:** *Check the answer you obtained for Question 7.5 by working through the calculation as described in Example 7:5.*

**ANSWER:** In the answer to Question 7.5 we stated that setting a 12.5 mg/20 mL solution at an infusion rate of 28.8 mL/hour would provide a dosage of 300 micrograms/minute.

Firstly, we need to calculate how much drug is administered per hour and then convert this to an administration rate per minute.

If there are 12.5 mg in every 20 mL of the infusion solution, in 28.8 mL, there would be:

$(12.5 \div 20) \times 28.8 = 18$ mg of drug.

This provides us with the amount of drug being administered per hour. Then this can be converted to an administration rate per minute.

$18 \div 60 = 0.3$ mg/min or 300 micrograms/min.

Therefore, a 12.5 mg/20 mL solution at an infusion rate of 28.8 mL/hour would provide a dosage of 300 micrograms/min.

**QUESTION 7.7:** *You are asked to calculate the amount of Drug E required to make 2.3 L of infusion where the administration rate is 5 mL/min and the dose is 60 microgram/kg/min. The patient weighs 80 kg.*

**ANSWER:**  Firstly, convert the dosage using the patient's weight:

If the dosage is 60 micrograms/kg/min and the patient weighs 80 kg, the dose is:

$60 \times 80 = 4800$ micrograms/min $\equiv 4.8$ mg/min.

If the administration rate is 5 mL/min and the dose is 4.8 mg/min, then the strength of the solution is 4.8 mg/5 mL.

Once we have calculated the strength of the solution, we can calculate the total quantity of Drug E for the required volume.

If there are 4.8 mg in every 5 mL, in 2.3 L (2300 mL) there are:

$(4.8 \div 5) \times 2300 = 2208$ mg.

Therefore, we require 2208 mg of Drug E to make 2.3 L of infusion where the administration rate is 5 mL/min and the dose is 60 micrograms/kg/min for an 80 kg patient.

---

**QUESTION 7.8:**  *Check the answer you obtained for Question 7.7 by working through the calculation as described in Example 7:8.*

**ANSWER:**  In the answer to Question 7.7 we stated that we would require 2208 mg of Drug E to make 2.3 L of infusion where the administration rate is 5 mL/min and the dose is 60 micrograms/kg/min for an 80 kg patient.

2208 mg of Drug E in 2300 mL would make:

$2208 \div 2300 = 0.96$ mg/mL $= 960$ micrograms/mL.

Then we can check the answer by either calculating the amount of drug to be administered per minute or the administration rate. First, calculate the amount of drug to be administered per minute.

If the solution contains 2208 mg of Drug E in every 2300 mL, in 5 mL (the amount administered per minute) there would be:

$(2208 \div 2300) \times 5 = 4.8$ mg/min.

To convert this to the original dose in micrograms/kg/min, we have to divide by the patient's weight. In this example, the patient weighs 80 kg.

$(4.8 \div 80) = 0.06$ mg/kg/min $\equiv 60$ micrograms/kg/min.

Alternatively, take the administration rate. If the dosage is 60 micrograms/kg/min and the patient weighs 80 kg, the dosage per minute is:

$60 \times 80 = 4800$ micrograms/min.

4800 micrograms/min would require an infusion rate (based on a solution concentration of 960 micrograms/mL) of:

$(4800 \div 960) = 5$ mL/min.

Therefore, 2208 mg of Drug E is required for a 2.3 L infusion where the administration rate is 5 mL/min and the dose is 60 micrograms/kg/min for an 80 kg patient.

**QUESTION 7.9:** *Calculate the volume of solution required (to two decimal places) for an infusion of Drug F, at a concentration of 65 mg/30 mL, where you are asked to infuse a total of 500 mg.*

**ANSWER:** If a total of 500 mg is to be infused, and the concentration of the desired solution is 65 mg/30 mL, the total volume required is:

$(30 \div 65) \times 500 = 230.77$ mL (to two decimal places).

Therefore, we will require a total of 230.77 mL (to two decimal places) of a 65 mg/30 mL solution of Drug F to infuse a total of 500 mg.

**QUESTION 7.10:** *At what rate (to two decimal places) would the infusion of Drug F from Question 7.9 need to be delivered to provide a dose of 7.5 mg/min? How long would the infusion last (to the nearest minute)?*

**ANSWER:** Firstly, calculate the infusion rate. If 7.5 mg/min is required, we need to know the volume of solution that contains 7.5 mg. As the solution is 65 mg/30 mL, this would be:

$(30 \div 65) \times 7.5 = 3.46$ mL/min (to two decimal places).

Next, we need to calculate how long the infusion will last. From the last calculation, we worked out that 3.46 mL of infusion would be administered every minute. Therefore, for 230.77 mL it would take:

$(230.77 \div 3.46) = 66.70$ min (to two decimal places) or 1 hour, 7 min (to the nearest minute).

Therefore, the infusion of Drug F from Question 7.9 would need to be delivered at 3.46 mL/min to provide a dose of 7.5 mg/min. The infusion would last a total of 1 hour, 7 min (to the nearest minute).

**QUESTION 7.11:** *An infusion of Drug G is to be delivered at a dose of 30 mg/kg/hour for 10 hours. After this time, the dose is reduced to 5 mg/kg/hour. How long would a 500 mL infusion bag at a concentration of 250 mg/1.5 mL last if the patient weighs 78 kg?*

**ANSWER:** To tackle this calculation we first need to work out how much drug will be required for the first 10 hours of infusion. If the dose is 30 mg/kg/hour and the patient weighs 78 kg, the amount of drug infused would be:

$30 \times 78 \times 10 = 23\,400$ mg (23.4 g).

Then we need to calculate the volume of infusion that this administration period would require. If there are 250 mg/1.5 mL, for 23 400 mg, we would infuse:

$(1.5 \div 250) \times 23\,400 = 140.4$ mL.

To work out how long the bag will last, we need to calculate the amount of time it will take to use the remainder of the bag after the infusion is reduced to an infusion rate of 5 mg/kg/hour. If the original bag was 500 mL and after 10 hours we have infused 140.4 mL, the remaining volume will be:

$500 - 140.4 = 359.6$ mL.

If there are 359.6 mL remaining and the bag has a concentration of 250 mg/1.5 mL, the amount of Drug G remaining is:

$(250 \div 1.5) \times 359.6 = 59\,933.33$ mg (to two decimal places).

At a (revised) administration rate of 5 mg/kg/hour and a patient weight of 78 kg, the revised rate per hour is:

$5 \times 78 = 390$ mg/hour.

Therefore, to use the remainder of Drug G (59 933.33 mg) it will take:

$59\,933.33 \div 390 = 153.68$ hours (to two decimal places) ≡ 153 hours, 41 min.

Therefore, in total, it will take:

$10 + 153.68 = 163.68$ hours (to two decimal places) ≡ 163 hours, 41 min.

---

**QUESTION 7.12:** *An infusion of Drug H is to be delivered at a dose of 35 mg/kg/hour for 3 hours. After this time, the dose is decreased to 20 mg/kg/hour. After the change of administration rate, how long (to the nearest minute) would it take for the remainder of a 1 L infusion bag at a concentration of 15 mg/mL to be administered if the patient weighs 65 kg?*

**ANSWER:** To tackle this calculation we first need to work out how much drug will be required for the first 3 hours of infusion. If the dose is 35 mg/kg/hour and the patient weighs 65 kg, the amount of drug infused would be:

$35 \times 65 \times 3 = 6825$ mg.

Then we need to calculate the volume of infusion that this administration period would require. If there are 15 mg/mL, for 6825 mg, we would infuse:

$(1 \div 15) \times 6825 = 455$ mL.

To work out how long the remainder of the bag will last, we need to calculate the amount of time it will take to use the remainder of the bag after the infusion is decreased to an infusion rate of 20 mg/kg/hour. If the original bag was 1 L (1000 mL) and after 3 hours we have infused 455 mL, the remaining volume will be:

$1000 - 455 = 545$ mL.

If there are 545 mL remaining and the bag has a concentration of 15 mg/mL, the amount of Drug H remaining is:

$(15 \div 1) \times 545 = 8175$ mg.

At a (revised) administration rate of 20 mg/kg/hour and a patient weight of 65 kg, the revised rate per hour is:

$20 \times 65 = 1300$ mg/hour.

Therefore, to use the remainder of Drug H (8175 mg) it will take:

$8175 \div 1300 = 6.29$ hours (to two decimal places) ≡ 6 hours, 17 min.

Therefore, after the end of the first administration period it will take a further 6 hours, 17 min (to the nearest minute) to administer the remainder of the infusion.

**QUESTION 7.13:** *A patient currently takes 35 mg of oral morphine twice a day (as sustained-release tablets). His doctor wants to change this to an intramuscular administration of diamorphine. What is the total daily dose of intramuscular diamorphine required? See* Prescribing in palliative care *within the current edition of the* British National Formulary *(and Example 7:13).*

**ANSWER:** To convert oral morphine to intramuscular diamorphine, you need to consult the equivalent dosage table in the *British National Formulary* (see *Prescribing in palliative care*). This states that the equivalent dose of intramuscular diamorphine is approximately one-third of the oral dose of morphine. Therefore, a twice-daily dose of 35 mg oral morphine is equivalent to:

$$(35 \times 2) \div 3 = 23.33 \text{ mg (to two decimal places)}.$$

Therefore, the total daily dose of intramuscular diamorphine required is 23.33 mg (to two decimal places).

**QUESTION 7.14:** *A patient currently takes 45 mg of oral morphine twice a day (as sustained-release tablets). Her doctor wants to change this to intramuscular administration. What is the dose of intramuscular morphine required? Note: see* Prescribing in palliative care *within the current edition of the* British National Formulary *(and Example 7:14).*

**ANSWER:** To convert oral morphine to intramuscular morphine, you need to halve the total daily dose and then divide into six (4-hourly) portions (see *Prescribing in palliative care* within the *British National Formulary*). Therefore, a twice-daily dose of 45 mg oral morphine is equivalent to a daily intramuscular dose of:

$$(45 \times 2) \div 2 = 45 \text{ mg}.$$

This would produce a 4-hourly dose of:

$$45 \div 6 = 7.5 \text{ mg}.$$

Therefore, the intramuscular morphine should be administered at a dose of 7.5 mg every 4 hours.

**QUESTION 7.15:** *A patient requires a dose of 45 mg/hour of Drug I. The solution in the syringe is 25 mg/5 mL and the syringe contains 50 mL and is 10 cm long. At what administration rate, in mm/hour, is the machine required to be set?*

**ANSWER:** Firstly, calculate the volume of drug required per hour. If the dose is 45 mg/hour and the solution is at a concentration of 25 mg/5 mL, the volume of drug required per hour is:

$$(5 \div 25) \times 45 = 9 \text{ mL/hour}.$$

Next, work out the length of the syringe which contains this volume. If we consider that the syringe is a fixed cylinder of 50 mL volume and 10 cm length, each cm of length is equivalent to:

$$50 \div 10 = 5 \text{ mL}.$$

Therefore, the required 9 mL will be the equivalent of:

$$9 \div 5 = 1.8 \text{ cm} \equiv 18 \text{ mm}.$$

This means that for a dose of 45 mg/hour of Drug I, a 50 mL syringe of 10 cm length containing a solution of 25 mg/5 mL needs to be set at an administration rate of 18 mm/hour.

**QUESTION 7.16:**   *A patient requires a dose of 270 mg/hour of Drug J. The solution in the infusion bag is 75 mg/10 mL and the bag contains 250 mL. The bag is set up on a giving set with a drop volume of 0.1 mL. At what drop rate (drops per minute) does the giving set need to be set?*

**ANSWER:**   Firstly, calculate the volume of drug required per minute. If the dose is 270 mg/hour and the solution is at a concentration of 75 mg/10 mL, the volume of drug required per hour is:

$(10 \div 75) \times 270 = 36$ mL/hour.

Next, convert this to a volume per minute.

$36 \div 60 = 0.6$ mL/minute.

Then convert this volume to drops based on each drop having a volume of 0.1 mL.

$0.6 \div 0.1 = 6$ drops/min.

Therefore, we need to set the giving set to 6 drops/min to provide a dose of 270 mg/hour of Drug J if the solution in the infusion bag is 75 mg/10 mL.

---

**QUESTION 7.17:**

*Roger has been admitted to hospital to enable his pain to be controlled. He has been taking one 30 mg sustained-release morphine tablet every 12 hours but his doctor wants to change him onto a subcutaneous dosage of diamorphine. With reference to the current British National Formulary, advise the doctor what the total daily dose of subcutaneous diamorphine would be.*

**ANSWER:**

To convert oral morphine to subcutaneous diamorphine, you need to consult the equivalent dosage table in the *British National Formulary* (see *Prescribing in palliative care*). This states that the equivalent dose of subcutaneous diamorphine is approximately one-third of the oral dose. Therefore, a twice-daily dose of 30 mg oral morphine is equivalent to:

$(30 \times 2) \div 3 = 20$ mg.

Therefore, the total daily dose of subcutaneous diamorphine required is 20 mg.

---

**QUESTION 7.18:**

*Geoff has been admitted to hospital and has been prescribed an antibiotic at 12 mg/kg/hour. The solution in the syringe is 250 mg/5 mL and the syringe contains 50 mL and is 10 cm long. At what administration rate, in mm/hour, is the machine required to be set?*

**ANSWER:**

Firstly, you need to convert Geoff's weight from stones and pounds to kilograms, noting that from previous calculations (see section 2.5.2) there are approximately 2.2 pounds in a kilogram. As Geoff weighs 12 stone and 6 pounds, his weight in pounds is:

$(12 \times 14) + 6 = 174$ pounds.

174 pounds in kilograms is:

$(174 \div 2.2) = 79.09$ kg (to two decimal places).

Next, calculate the volume of drug required per hour. If the dose is 12 mg/kg/hour and the solution is at a concentration of 250 mg/5 mL, the volume of drug required per hour is:

$(5 \div 250) \times (12 \times 79.09) = 18.98$ mL/hour (to two decimal places).

Next, work out the length of the syringe that contains this volume. If we consider that the syringe is a fixed cylinder of 50 mL volume and 10 cm length, each cm of length is equivalent to:

$50 \div 10 = 5$ mL.

Therefore, the required 18.98 mL will be the equivalent of:

$18.98 \div 5 = 3.80$ cm (to two decimal places).

This means that for a dose of 12 mg/kg/hour of that antibiotic, a 50 mL syringe of 10 cm length containing a solution of 250 mg/5 mL needs to be set at an administration rate of 38 mm/hour.

# Data: presentation, interpretation, and basic statistics

# 8

## 8.1 Chapter introduction

As a pharmacist it is necessary to understand the concepts of data presentation and data analysis. Within this chapter we explore the graphical presentation of data, and how we can use such graphs to mathematically represent the data. Although linear relationships are easy to represent with straight-line plots, not all data will fit such plots. Therefore, methods to plot data in such a way that we can form a straight line are outlined. These processes are then applied to considering the stability of medicines. Within this chapter, we also introduce basic statistics. This helps us analyse and make decisions on data collected from research projects, or data collected at an advanced level, such as from clinical trials. An understanding of basic statistics also helps in the critical evaluation of published research that can influence patient care and improvements in healthcare provision. This is particularly important as statistics can be used and abused, so a working knowledge of basic statistics is a useful tool; it allows us to compare data sets and make predictions from data.

## 8.2 Presentation of data using tables and graphs

To interpret data and find patterns in data sets we need to be able to present collected data. The first step in collecting data is generally to tabulate it, then to plot the data values as points on a graph. There are two main categories of graphs used in the presentation of scientific data:

1. Graphs used to describe the relationship between variables.
2. Graphs employed to show the distribution of data.

### 8.2.1 Graphs describing the relationship between variables

When using graphs to describe the relationship between variables, the first step is to consider which variable is the dependent variable and which is the independent variable. The independent variable comprises the values chosen by the experimenter. For example when considering drug release from a tablet over time, time would be the independent variable. Alternatively, when considering the number of obese patients living within a geographical area, the geographical area is the independent variable. In both these studies, the other variable (i.e. drug release and number of obese patients) is the dependent variable, as these values depend on the choice for the independent variable.

| **EXAMPLE 8:1** | |
|---|---|
| **Question:** | Identify the independent variable in each of the following experiments.<br><br>a) Plasma drug concentration measured over time.<br><br>b) The viscosity of an ointment at different temperatures.<br><br>c) The effect of a new drug dose on blood pressure. |
| **Answer:** | a) Time.<br><br>b) Temperature.<br><br>c) Drug dose. |

In a typical experiment, the researcher will allow the independent variable to change (normally to increase, but decreasing the independent variable is also an option) at regular intervals and the dependent variable will be measured. The results are then tabulated with the independent variable on the left, and the dependent variable on the right. The table shows us the data, but it is difficult for us to interpret the data and see any trends. However, we can interpret the data by plotting a graph. There are a range of options that may be used to plot relationships between data, for example scatter graphs, line graphs, and bar graphs. Of these options, scatter graphs are generally the most useful for displaying a correlation between data. Below are the key basic rules for plotting a scatter graph:

- Draw the horizontal x-axis for the values of the independent variable (the variable the researcher has set).
- Draw the vertical y-axis for the values of the dependent variable (the variable the researcher has measured).
- Use suitable scales on each axis, so that the data can be easily visualized; this will depend on the end-values for your data points.
- Label each axis with the variable and its units.
- If the graph contains two or more plots, a key that identifies the symbols of each plot should be provided.
- It is often important to include estimates of variability in data in graphs using error bars. Here it is important to note which estimate of variability has been used, for example standard deviation or standard error.

When we plot data we are often looking for a trend or a general correlation between the factors plotted. Figure 8.1 shows three graphs, each with a different type of relationship between the dependent and independent variable.

Figure 8.1(a) shows a schematic of a straight-line graph, which passes through the origin. Figure 8.1(b) shows there is a relationship between the two variables, where y is decreasing with x, but we do not have a linear correlation. Figure 8.1(c) depicts a graph where no relationship is apparent between the two variables.

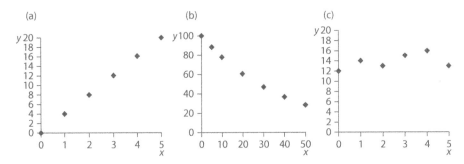

**Figure 8.1** Graphs with and without relationships between the dependent and independent variable.

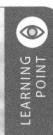

### Plotting a graph to describe the relationship between variables

Plotting data on a graph can show relationships between the variables plotted. When plotting data be sure to use suitable scales on your axes and appropriate labels. Scatter plots are useful for considering if there is a linear relationship between the dependent and independent variables.

LEARNING POINT

## 8.2.2 Graphs used to show data distribution

Graphs can also be employed to describe the distribution of data; histograms and dot-plots are both types of graph that define the frequency of distribution of data. Frequency distributions are commonly employed to consider the shape of the data distribution. In these graphs, the data are divided up into intervals and then presented as the number of observations that fall into each interval. For example, this could include plotting student exam grades where the data are divided up into categories 10 points wide (e.g. 0-10, 10-20, 20-30, etc.) on the x-axis, and the y-axis indicates the number of students getting a grade within this range. Alternatively this could be used to plot the size distribution of particles within a suspension, with size ranges presented on the x-axis and the percentage of the particle population within each size range shown on the y-axis. This can be useful as it gives an indication of the distribution of particle sizes and potential bimodal distribution.

Alternative options for presenting data include the use of pie charts, which can be good for comparing the relative contribution that different categories contribute to an overall total. Pie charts often present data in the form of percentages. These types of charts give a good visualization of the data when the categories show variation in size. Generally, they are effective when displaying data for up to around six categories. Above this, they can become difficult to read and a table or bar graph may be more effective.

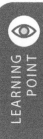

**Plotting a graph to show the distribution of data**

Histograms and dot-plots can be used to display the frequency distribution of data. In these, the horizontal scale represents the characteristic measured and the vertical axis indicates the corresponding frequency of occurrence (generally in per cent).

Pie charts give a visual representation to show proportions of a total amount, for example the number of students getting a 1st, 2:1, 2:2, and 3rd in their MPharm degree.

## 8.3 Linear and logarithmic calculations

If there is a linear relationship between the variables plotted, that is we can put a straight line through a set of data points, then this linear relationship is represented by the equation of the line in the form $y=mx+c$ (see Figure 8.2).

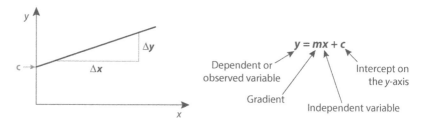

**Figure 8.2** Linear relationship graph of $y=mx+c$.

Any equation in the format of $y=mx+c$ that involves multiples of $x$ (e.g. $y=2x+6$) but no higher powers (such as $x^2$) follows a linear relationship. It is easy to determine the equation of a straight line and use this to calculate data from incomplete data sets. To obtain the equation for the line, '$c$' is the intercept of the graph on the $y$-axis, and $m$ is the gradient of the line. We can calculate $m$ using the following equation:

$$m = \frac{change\ in\ y}{change\ in\ x} = \frac{y_2 - y_1}{x_2 - x_1} = \frac{\Delta y}{\Delta x}$$

Therefore, if the data can be fitted to this form, and we have this equation, for any value of $x$, then we can calculate the value of $y$. Commonly, computer packages, such as Microsoft Excel or Graphpad Prism, are used to prepare graphs with the option of displaying the equation of the line. By plotting data and obtaining the relationship between data this allows for **interpolation** and **extrapolation** of data.

- Interpolation allows for values in between known data points to be estimated.

- Extrapolation estimates the values beyond the available range of information.

Both of these processes do have associated assumptions in that all the data fits the graph and that the correlation of the data continues beyond the measured values, which may not be the case. However through this process, we can estimate the value of the dependent value if we know the independent value.

**EXAMPLE 8:2**

**Question:** Deduce the equation of the lines from the following information.

a) The gradient of the line is 10 and the line passes through the y-axis at 8.

b) The gradient of the line is $-4$ and the line passes through the y-axis at $-12$.

**Answer:**

a) $y = 10x + 8$.

b) $y = -4x - 12$.

**EXAMPLE 8:3**

**Question:** Varying amounts of drug were dissolved in water and the optical absorbance of each solution has been measured. Plot the data and obtain the equation of the line. Use the equation of the line to calculate the drug concentration of a solution that has a UV absorbance of 0.650.

| Drug concentration (mg/dm³) | UV absorption |
|---|---|
| 0 | 0.002 |
| 20 | 0.267 |
| 40 | 0.583 |
| 60 | 0.824 |
| 80 | 1.120 |
| 100 | 1.313 |

**Answer:**

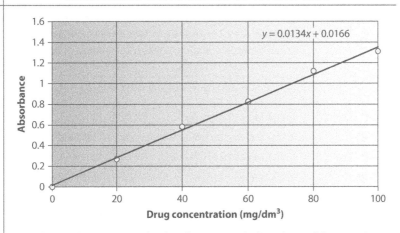

$y = 0.0134x + 0.0166$

From the graph, we can see the data fit to a straight-line plot and the equation of the line shows that the intercept is 0.0166 and the gradient is 0.0134.

The concentration of a drug solution with a UV absorbance of 0.650 is calculated as follows:

$y$ = UV absorbance of the drug solution = 0.650.

$x$ = drug concentration.

Therefore $0.650 = 0.0134x + 0.0166$.

$0.0134x = 0.650 - 0.0166$.

$x = 47 \, \text{mg/dm}^3$.

Therefore, the drug concentration of the solution is 47 mg/dm³.

### 8.3.1 Determining the equation of a straight line from limited data

Sometimes we may not have the graph, but if we have the gradient of the straight line (or the rate of change) and a single point that lies on the line, we can calculate the equation of the straight line. Alternatively if we have only two points from the straight line, but not the gradient, the equation of the line can be calculated.

| EXAMPLE 8:4 | |
|---|---|
| **Question:** | Deduce the equation of the straight line given that the gradient of the line is 2.5 and the line passes through the point (4, 5). |
| **Answer:** | The equation of the line is: $y = mx + c$ and $m = 2.5$. |
| | Therefore $y = 2.5x + c$; however, we still need to calculate $c$, and we know when $x = 4$, $y = 5$. So we can add these values into the equation: |
| | $5 = (2.5 \times 4) + c$, and thus $c = -5$. |
| | Therefore the equation of the line is $y = 2.5x - 5$. |

| EXAMPLE 8:5 | |
|---|---|
| **Question:** | Dr Walter White designs a production process that produces 15 kg of new drug per hour. After 1 hour, the production plant contains a total of 40 kg of the drug. Write an equation to relate the amount of new drug in the production plant and the process time, assuming no drug is removed. |
| **Answer:** | Start by defining the terms; we have two variables, the amount of drug produced and the time of the process. $y$ is the amount of drug in the production plant and $x$ is the process time. We also know the rate of production is 15 kg per hour, so we equate the rate with the gradient $m$. |
| | The equation of the line is: $y = mx + c$ and $m = 15$ kg per hour. |
| | Therefore: $y = 15x + c$; however, we still need to calculate $c$. |
| | In the above example, after 1 hour, 15 kg of drug is produced and we have a total of 40 kg of new drug in the production plant, so: |
| | $40 = (15 \times 1) + c$, and thus $c = 25$. |
| | Therefore the equation of the line is $y = 15x + 25$. |

| | EXAMPLE 8:6 |
|---|---|
| Question: | Two points on the calibration line of an absorbance (y) vs concentration (x) graph are:<br><br>• 20 mg/mL, absorbance = 0.4.<br>• 40mg/mL, absorbance = 0.8.<br><br>Calculate the equation of the line and the concentration equivalent to an absorbance of 0.7. |
| Answer: | $m = \dfrac{change\ in\ y}{change\ in\ x} = \dfrac{y_2 - y_1}{x_2 - x_1} = \dfrac{\Delta y}{\Delta x}$<br><br>$m = \dfrac{0.8 - 0.4}{40 - 20}$<br><br>$m = 0.02.$<br><br>The equation of the line is: $y = mx + c$ and $m = 0.02$.<br><br>Therefore, $y = 0.02x + c$; however, we still need to calculate $c$.<br><br>You can use either of the data sets for the two points for $x$ and $y$:<br><br>$c = 0.8 - (0.02 \times 40).$<br><br>$c = 0$, and the equation of the line is $y = 0.02x$<br><br>To calculate the concentration equivalent to an absorbance of 0.7:<br><br>$y = 0.02x.$<br><br>Therefore, $0.7 = 0.02x.$<br><br>$x = 35\ mg/mL.$ |

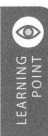

## Calculating a linear relationship

With the gradient of a straight line (or the rate of change) and a single point that lies on the line, we can calculate the equation of the straight line. This will give us the relationship between x and y. Alternatively, if we have only two points from the straight line, we can calculate the gradient and then the equation of the line.

LEARNING POINT

### 8.3.2 Obtaining straight-line graphs from non-linear functions

Although linear relationships are easy to represent with straight-line plots, not all data will fit such plots. This can occur in a range of situations, for example radioactive decay, bacterial growth, and chemical reaction kinetics. The lack of linearity does not mean there is no relationship between the data; data-plotting packages, such as Excel, can give the equation of a range of plots. However, sometimes working with a curved line can be more difficult than handling a straight-line plot. To address this, there are methods to plot data in such a way that we can form a straight line, that is we can linearize the plot. Then, when we have a straight-line graph, we can determine its gradient and intercept as outlined previously.

### 8.3.2.1 Log linearization

We know that any linear equation with two variables can be written in the form $y = mx + c$, and that its graph will be a straight line. Graphs that contain power function: $y = kx^m$ and $y = km^x$ (where $x$ is the independent variable, $y$ is the dependent variable, and $k$ and $m$ are constants) will give curved graphs; however, we can convert these graphs into straight-line plots using logarithmic functions (either ln or log). This then gives us straight-line graphs, which are easier to deal with than curves, and we can measure the gradient and the intercept to define the line.

Using logs, this is achieved as follows:

$$y = kx^m$$

$$log(y) = log(kx^m)$$

$$log(y) = log(k) + log(x^m)$$

$$log(y) = log(k) + mlog(x)$$

Then the data when plotted convert from a curve to a straight-line graph, where $m$ represents the gradient and $log(k)$ the intercept (Figure 8.3).

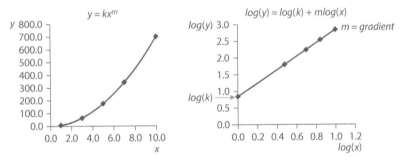

**Figure 8.3** Log linearization of data that fit the equation $y = kx^m$.

A similar principle can be applied to linearize exponential equations of the type $y = km^x$. The log linearization is as follows:

$$y = km^x$$

$$log(y) = log(km^x)$$

$$log(y) = log(k) + log(m^x)$$

$$log(y) = log(k) + xlog(m)$$

However in this case, $x$ is not a log, therefore we plot $log(y)$ against $x$ to get a straight line where $log(m)$ represents the gradient and $log(k)$ the intercept (Figure 8.4).

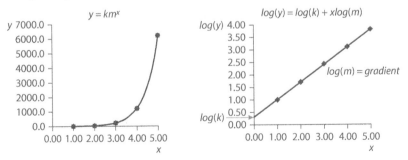

**Figure 8.4** Log linearization of data that fit the equation $y = km^x$.

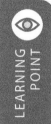

## Rules for handling ln and logs

$log(a.b) = log(a) + log(b)$

$log(a/b) = log(a) - log(b)$

$log(a^b) = b.log(a)$

$log(k.a^b) = log(k) + b.log(a)$

The natural logarithm of a number is its logarithm to the base $e$. The rules for handling logs also apply to natural logs. The natural log of $e$, that is to say $ln(e) = 1$.

LEARNING POINT

| | EXAMPLE 8:7 |
|---|---|
| **Question:** | Log linearize the following equation of a curve: $y = 5x^2$. From this linearized equation, what would be the intercept and the gradient of the line? |
| **Answer:** | $y = 5x^2$ <br><br> $log(y) = log(5x^2)$ <br><br> $log(y) = log(5) + log(x^2)$ <br><br> $log(y) = 0.70 + 2log(x)$ <br><br> Therefore, the gradient would be 2 and the intercept would be $log(5) = 0.70$. |

| | EXAMPLE 8:8 |
|---|---|
| **Question:** | Log linearize the following equation of a curve: $y = 2^x$. From this linearized equation, what would be the intercept and the gradient of the line? |
| **Answer:** | $y = 2^x$ <br><br> $log(y) = log(2^x)$ <br><br> $log(y) = xlog(2)$ <br><br> $log(y) = 0.3x$ <br><br> Therefore, the gradient would be $log(2) = 0.30$ and the intercept $= 0$. |

| | EXAMPLE 8:9 |
|---|---|
| **Question:** | You are presented with the following data from an experiment considering the concentration of benzocaine in solution over time. When these data are plotted, the following graph is obtained. Use log linearization of the data and calculate the gradient and intercept of the line from this equation. |

| Time (days) | Benzocaine concentration (mmol/L) |
|-------------|-----------------------------------|
| 0 | 100.0 |
| 5 | 88.25 |
| 10 | 77.90 |
| 20 | 60.65 |
| 30 | 47.25 |
| 40 | 36.80 |
| 50 | 28.65 |

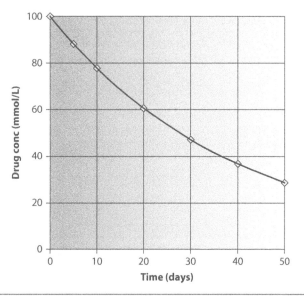

**Answer:** By taking the log of the drug concentration, and plotting log y against x, a straight-line graph is produced and both the gradient ($-0.01$) and the intercept (2.00) can be calculated.

| Time (days) | Benzocaine concentration (mmol/L) | log (drug conc) |
|-------------|-----------------------------------|-----------------|
| 0 | 100.00 | 2.00 |
| 5 | 88.25 | 1.95 |
| 10 | 77.90 | 1.89 |
| 20 | 60.65 | 1.78 |
| 30 | 47.25 | 1.67 |
| 40 | 36.80 | 1.57 |
| 50 | 28.65 | 1.46 |

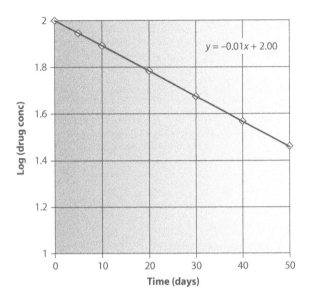

### 8.3.2.2 Using natural logs

The same can be achieved using the natural log, ln. This is particularly useful when dealing with exponential functions ($e^x$) and commonly used in first order reaction kinetics where the concentration decreases with time as follows:

$$C_t = C_0 e^{-kt}$$

Where $C_0$ = initial concentration, $C_t$ = concentration after time $t$, $t$ = time, $k$ = rate constant.

To linearize this expression, take natural logs (ln) (remember $\ln(e) = 1$) (see Figure 8.5).

$$\ln C_t = \ln C_0 - k.t$$

Thus you can convert values of $C_t$ to $\ln C_t$ and the plot of $\ln C_t$ (y-axis) against t (x-axis) gives a straight line with a slope of –k (i.e. negative) and an intercept of $\ln C_0$ (Figure 8.5). Alternatively, data can be plotted on semi-log paper to produce a straight-line plot.

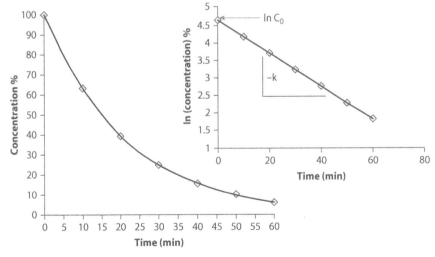

**Figure 8.5** Natural log linearization of data fitting the equation $C_t = C_0 e^{-kt}$.

| | **EXAMPLE 8:10** |
|---|---|
| **Question:** | Use natural logs to linearize the following equations. |
| | $y = 8e^x$. |
| | $y = e^{-21x}$. |
| | $C_t = C_0 e^{-kt}$. |
| | $C_t = 5e^{-7t}$. |
| **Answer:** | $ln(y) = ln(8) + xln(e)$, therefore, $ln(y) = 2.08 + x$ (remember $ln(e) = 1$). |
| | $ln(y) = -21x$. |
| | $ln(C_t) = ln(C_0) - kt$. |
| | $ln(C_t) = ln(5) - 7t$, therefore, $ln(C_t) = 1.61 - 7t$. |

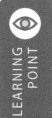

### Summary of key equations

The equation of a straight line: $y = mx + c$.

If a line has the form, $y = kx^m$, then $log(y) = log(k) + mlog(x)$.

Plotting $log(y)$ on the y-axis and $log(x)$ on the x-axis will give you a straight-line plot where $m$ is the gradient and $log(k)$ is the intercept.

If a line has the form $y = km^x$, then $log(y) = log(k) + xlog(m)$

Plotting $log(y)$ on the y-axis and $x$ on the x-axis, will give you a straight-line plot where $log(m)$ is the gradient and $log(k)$ is the intercept.

Remember these rules apply for both log and ln.

**LEARNING POINT**

## 8.4 Stability of medicines

A key factor in the stability of medicines is drug degradation. Degradation, like any reaction process may follow zero order, first order, pseudo-first order, or second order kinetics. The order of the reaction is the number of concentration terms that determine the rate of reaction. Degradation of a drug may follow zero order kinetics if the concentration of the drug in solution does not influence the rate of the reaction (i.e. the rate of reaction is independent of the concentration of the reactants):

$$C_t = C_0 - k_0 t$$

For first order reactions, the concentration of the drug remaining at time t ($C_t$) is dependent on the initial drug concentration and the reaction rate constant:

$$C_t = C_0 . e^{-kt}$$

This can be written in its linearized format as (see section 8.3.2.2):

$$\ln C_t = \ln C_0 - k.t$$

In both equations:

$C_0$ = initial concentration, $C_t$ = concentration after time t, t = time, k = rate constant.

Plotting drug concentration against time can give you an indication of the order of the reaction. If the concentration of drug against time plot is linear, this indicates zero order reaction kinetics (Figure 8.6(a)). If a plot of ln(drug concentration) against time gives a straight-line plot this indicates a first order reaction process for degradation (Figure 8.6(b)). From these plots we can calculate both the order of the reaction and the rate constant, which can then be used to calculate drug concentration at a given time point.

(a) Zero order reaction: $C_t = C_0 - k_0 t$

(b) First order: $\ln(C_t) = \ln(C_0) - k_1 t$

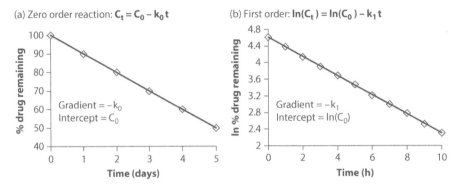

Figure 8.6 Zero and first order drug degradation reactions.

---

**EXAMPLE 8:11**

**Question:** The data given below represent the hydrolysis of a drug over time. Calculate the order of reaction and the rate constant.

| Time (days) | Drug concentration (mg/mL) |
|---|---|
| 0 | 19.8 |
| 1 | 16.6 |
| 2 | 12.8 |
| 3 | 9.2 |
| 4 | 5.5 |
| 5 | 1.9 |

**Answer:** First plot the data on a graph of concentration against time:

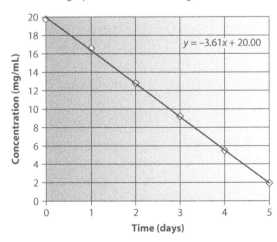

As the data are a straight-line plot of $C_t$ against time, this means the degradation follows zero order kinetics. From the graph, the gradient is $-3.61$. The gradient $= -k_0$, therefore $k_0 = 3.61$.

| EXAMPLE 8:12 | |
|---|---|
| **Question:** | To investigate the stability of a drug in solution, the drug concentration is measured over time. The degradation process is shown to follow zero order kinetics. If the initial drug concentration is 100 mg/mL, what concentration will be remaining after 3 days if the rate constant $k_0 = 2.30 \, \text{day}^{-1}$? |
| **Answer:** | $C_t = C_0 - k_0 t$. <br> $C_t = 100 \, \text{mg/mL} - (2.30 \times 3)$. <br> $C_t = 93.1 \, \text{mg/mL}$. |

| EXAMPLE 8:13 | |
|---|---|
| **Question:** | A drug is shown to degrade by first order rate kinetics. If the rate constant $k_1 = 0.002 \, \text{day}^{-1}$, what percentage of drug will remain after 10 days? |
| **Answer:** | $\ln C_t = \ln C_0 - k_1 t$. <br> $\ln C_t = \ln 100 - (0.002 \times 10)$. <br> $\ln C_t = 4.61 - 0.02 = 4.59$. <br> $C_t = 98\%$, therefore 98% of the drug will be remaining after 10 days. |

**Stability of medicines**

Drug degradation may follow zero order kinetics:

$$C_t = C_0 - k_0 t$$

Or first order kinetics:

$$\ln C_t = \ln C_0 - k_1 t$$

Where $C_0 =$ initial concentration, $C_t =$ concentration after time t, t = time, k = rate constant.

Plotting drug concentration against time can give you an indication of the order of the reaction.

LEARNING POINT

### 8.4.1 Overage

Given that degradation of a drug on storage leads to a decline in potency, adding excess of an active ingredient can overcome this problem; this is known as 'overage', where additional drug is added to maintain the drug concentration within therapeutic limits for a specified time. In such a process, consideration of the break-down products must be given and overage is not commonly used. However, by using the degradation profile (rate constant and rate of reaction), an overage can be calculated to ensure the concentration of a drug after a set period. It is important not to confuse this with the same term that is used when we supply more of a medicine than required to allow for loss during administration (e.g. supplying an overage of a liquid medication to allow for any loss caused by transference during measurement of each of the individual dosages).

| **EXAMPLE 8:14** | |
|---|---|
| **Question:** | In Example 8.12 calculate the overage required to ensure a drug concentration of 95 mg/mL after 5 days. |
| **Answer:** | In this instance we know we want $C_t = 95$ mg/mL after 5 days, so we need to identify what the starting concentration ($C_0$) should be. <br><br> $C_t = C_0 - k_0 t$ <br><br> $95 \, \text{mg/mL} = C_0 - (2.30 \times 5)$. <br><br> $C_0 = 95 + 11.5 \, \text{mg/mL} = 106.5 \, \text{mg/mL}$. <br><br> Therefore, an overage of 6.5 mg/mL is required. |

## Overage

Overage can consider the addition of drug to a formulation to achieve a drug concentration at a specified time. The overage required can be calculated if the rate constant is known and the order of reaction kinetics.

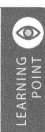

LEARNING POINT

### 8.4.2 Shelf-life and the effect of temperature

The shelf-life of a medical product is the time that the required drug characteristics (e.g. potency) remain within an approved specification after manufacture. An expiration date is the termination of shelf-life, and after this time the medicine may no longer function as intended. The shelf-life is assessed as the length of time required for the product specifications to be reduced to some percentage of the original value. For most products, this is the time at which the products retain 90% of the original potency. A range of factors can influence product stability, including temperature, humidity, light, and oxygen. Drug products degrade by several different types of reactions and it is important to monitor several product attributes in addition to the main drug content including:

- Physical attributes, for example particle size, appearance.
- Chemical attributes, for example drug assay, degradants, pH.

- In vitro drug release rate/dissolution.
- Biological attributes, for example bioassay and microbial attributes.

The shelf-life is established by conducting stability tests in accordance with prescribed protocols. A selection of samples, from a range of batches of a product, are stored at defined storage conditions. These can include:

- Long-term stability: the product is held at 25°C and 60% relative humidity.
- Intermediate conditions: 30°C and 65% relative humidity.
- Accelerated conditions: 40°C and 75% relative humidity.
- Stress conditions, for example light, acid, oxidative conditions.

Although drug stability at room temperature is of primary interest, measuring this can be a lengthy process. Therefore, accelerated conditions involving storage at elevated temperatures can be used in accordance with the Arrhenius equation, which is a formula for the temperature dependence of reaction rates:

$$k = Ae^{-\frac{E_A}{RT}}$$

Where k = rate constant of a chemical reaction, A = the Arrhenius factor or the frequency factor, R = the gas constant, $E_A$ = the activation energy, T = temperature in Kelvin.

Using log linearization we can write this equation as:

$$\ln k = \ln A - \frac{E_A}{RT}$$

This form of the equation now fits the general equation for a straight line ($y = mx + c$), and a plot of ln k against 1/T has a gradient of $-E_A/R$ (see Figure 8.7).

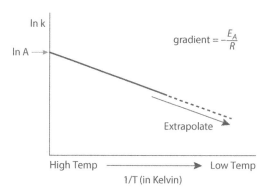

**Figure 8.7** The Arrhenius plot showing the variation of ln k with 1/T.

Therefore, the Arrhenius equation can be used to predict the reaction rates at storage temperatures from data at high temperatures, as we can extrapolate from the higher temperature results and use the straight-line plot to calculate the rate constant of the reaction at a given temperature. Given that most reaction rates increase by temperature, increased temperatures can be used to plot ln k against 1/T (a generalization supported by the Arrhenius equation is that for many common chemical reactions at room temperature, the reaction rate doubles for every 10°C increase in temperature). From this, k at a given temperature (e.g. 25°C for shelf-life calculations) can be calculated. Using this, we can calculate the shelf-life of a product.

**EXAMPLE 8:15**

**Question:** From the following data, estimate the rate constant of a new drug solution at 25°C. Calculate the shelf-life of the drug solution at 25°C, assuming the degradation of the drug follows first order reaction kinetics where the concentration decreases with time as follows: $\ln C_t = \ln C_0 - k.t.$

| Temperature (°C) | k (day⁻¹) |
|---|---|
| 70 | 0.0392 |
| 60 | 0.0164 |
| 50 | 0.0056 |
| 40 | 0.0022 |

**Answer:** First we need to calculate 1/T (in Kelvin) and ln k.

| Temperature (°C) | k (day⁻¹) | T(K) | 1/T | ln k |
|---|---|---|---|---|
| 70 | 0.0392 | 343 | 0.0029 | −3.24 |
| 60 | 0.0164 | 333 | 0.0030 | −4.11 |
| 50 | 0.0056 | 323 | 0.0031 | −5.18 |
| 40 | 0.0022 | 313 | 0.0032 | −6.12 |

Then we plot ln k against 1/T and calculate the equation of the line:

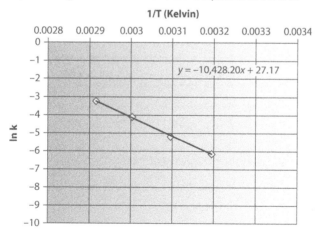

From this we can now calculate k at 25°C (298K):

$\ln k = 27.17 - 10\,428.20/T.$

$\ln k = 27.17 - 34.99 = -7.82.$

Therefore $k = 0.0004$ (this can also be done by extrapolation of the line).

At a shelf-life of 90% of the stated active ingredient remaining:

$C_t = C_0 \cdot e^{-kt}$, where $C_t$ = drug concentration at 90%, $C_0$ is 100%, and k we have calculated at 25°C.

Therefore:

$\ln C_t = \ln C_0 - k.t.$

$$t = \frac{\ln(\frac{C_0}{C_t})}{k} = \frac{\ln(\frac{100}{90})}{0.0004} = 263 \text{ days.}$$

Therefore, the shelf-life of the product is 263 days at 25°C.

In section 8.3.1, it was shown how the equation of a line can be derived from two data points assuming that the data follow a straight-line plot. This can be applied to the calculation of shelf-life.

---

**EXAMPLE 8:16**

**Question:** From the following data, estimate the rate constant of a new drug solution at 25°C. Calculate the shelf-life of the drug solution at 25°C, assuming the degradation of the drug follows first order reaction kinetics where the concentration decreases with time as follows: $\ln C_t = \ln C_0 - k.t.$

| Temperature (°C) | k (day$^{-1}$) |
|---|---|
| 60 | 0.008 |
| 40 | 0.001 |

**Answer:** First we need to calculate 1/T (in Kelvin) and ln k.

| Temperature (°C) | k (day$^{-1}$) | T(K) | 1/T | ln k |
|---|---|---|---|---|
| 60 | 0.008 | 333 | 0.0030 | -4.83 |
| 40 | 0.001 | 313 | 0.0032 | -6.91 |

The gradient is calculated as:

$$m = \frac{change\ in\ y}{change\ in\ x} = \frac{y_2 - y_1}{x_2 - x_1} = \frac{\Delta y}{\Delta x}$$

$= (-4.83 - (-6.91)) \div (0.0030 - 0.0032).$

$= 2.08 \div (-0.0002) = -10400.$

The equation of the line is: $y = mx + c$ and $m = -10400$, therefore:

$-4.83 = (-10400*0.0030) + c.$

$c = 31.2 - 4.83 = 26.4.$

From this we can now calculate k at 25°C (298K):

$\ln k = 26.4 - 10400/T$.

$\ln k = 26.4 - 34.9 = -8.5$.

Therefore $k = 0.0002$.

At a shelf-life of 90% of the stated active ingredient remaining:

$C_t = C_0 . e^{-kt}$, where $C_t$ = drug concentration at 90%, $C_0$ is 100%, and k we have calculated at 25°C. Therefore:

$\ln C_t = \ln C_0 - k.t$.

$$t = \frac{\ln(\frac{C_0}{C_t})}{k} = \frac{\ln(\frac{100}{90})}{0.0002} = 527 \text{ days}.$$

Therefore the shelf-life of the product is 527 days at 25°C.

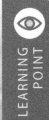

**Arrhenius equation**

The Arrhenius equation can be used to predict the reaction rates at storage temperatures. Using this, the shelf-life of a product can be calculated:

$$k = Ae^{-\frac{E_A}{RT}}$$

Using log linearization we can write this equation as:

$$\ln k = \ln A - \frac{E_A}{RT}$$

Where k = rate constant of a chemical reaction, A = the Arrhenius factor or the frequency factor, R = the gas constant, $E_A$ = the activation energy, T = temperature in Kelvin.

LEARNING POINT

### 8.4.3 Half-life

The half-life of a reaction is the time taken for the initial concentration to fall by half. Therefore in this instance $C_t$ is set at 50% (rather than 90% as it was in the above examples). As before, the half-life can follow zero or first order kinetics.

## 8.5 Simple statistics: analysis of data

Statistics is an important tool; it allows us to summarize experimental data in terms of the central tendency (mean and median) and variance (standard deviation, standard error of the mean, range and confidence interval) as shown in Chapter 3. It also enables us to consider whether data sets are different from each other, for example when considering if the pharmacological effect of one drug is superior to another, or if a drug is making a difference on a clinical outcome. Therefore, it is vital we understand statistics. To cover this topic in detail is beyond the scope of this book, however, and readers are referred to other texts for further development of their statistical understanding[9].

9 For example, Jones, D (2002). *Pharmaceutical Statistics*, Pharmaceutical Press, UK.

Nonetheless, an overview of statistical testing to measure whether differences in data sets are meaningful is useful both in the consideration of experimental designs and for critical evaluation of data and published research.

### 8.5.1 Calculating confidence intervals

In Chapter 3, the concept of calculating the mean and measuring the variability of data was outlined. This gave a method by which a data set could be summarized and the variability within the data set represented. As discussed, experimental data sets are normally a sample from a population and it is important to consider if these sample data are a good representation of the population data. To do this we need an indicator of the reliability of this data. That is to say, we need a measure of how confident we are that this sample data set will contain the true mean value. This is achieved by using **confidence intervals** that give the probability that a sample of data will contain the true mean. For example, in considering the average height of men in England, it would be laborious to obtain the height of all men, therefore, we could take a random sample of men from the population and find the mean height from this sample of men. It would be expected that the mean height from a sample would be close, but not equal to the mean height of the entire population. The confidence interval would tell us the probability that the sample height data collected would contain the true mean height for the population. Basically, confidence intervals provide a range which we know is likely to contain the true, but unknown, mean. Clearly, if you already knew the population mean, there would be no need for a confidence interval. The end points of the confidence interval are called the confidence limits.

With data sets, the user sets confidence intervals and most commonly the confidence intervals are set at 95% and they are quoted as the mean of the data set and the confidence interval. If we have a confidence interval of 90%, there is a 90% chance that the true mean will lie within the calculated range. Similarly, if we have a 99% confidence interval, there is a 99% chance that the true mean will be within the calculated range. These confidence intervals are related to the standard errors as follows (Figure 8.8):

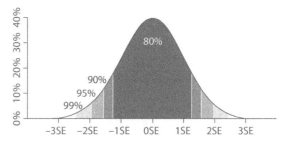

**Figure 8.8** Sampling distribution of means.

- 90% of sample means lie within ± 1.64 standard errors of the population mean.
- 95% of sample means lie within ± 1.96 standard errors of the population mean.
- 99% of sample means lie within ± 2.58 standard errors of the population mean.

Within Figure 8.8, the scale on the x-axis is the number of standard errors and the shaded portions show the proportion of data. Therefore to cover 99% of the data, you include all shaded portions. To cover 80%, you include the darkest blue section only.

Alternatively, we can consider that the confidence interval provides a range for our best guess of the size of the population mean that is plausible given the size of the sample mean. To calculate the confidence intervals for data that conform to a normal distribution, the following equation is used:

$$\text{confidence interval} = \text{mean} \pm Z_{p\%} (\text{SEM}).$$

The $Z_{p\%}$ is a value dependent on the confidence interval being calculated. For a confidence interval of:

$$90\%, Z_{p\%} = 1.65.$$

$$95\%, Z_{p\%} = 1.96.$$

$$99\%, Z_{p\%} = 2.58.$$

However, a confidence interval of 95% is commonly used as it is narrow enough to be informative but is seldom misleading. With this we are saying we can be 95% confident that any sample mean measured is going to be within plus or minus 1.96 standard errors of the population mean. Remember the standard error is dependent on the standard deviation and the size of the sample (a small standard deviation gives a small standard error, and a small sample size gives a large standard error).

---

**EXAMPLE 8:17**

**Question:** The average plasma drug concentration in patients in a clinical trial, where the sample size (n) is 106, was $61.6 \pm 10.9$ micrograms/mL (mean $\pm$ SD). Calculate the 90%, 95%, and 99% confidence intervals assuming the data originated from a normal distribution.

**Answer:** First you calculate the standard error of the mean (as outlined in Chapter 3):

$$\text{Standard error} = \frac{\text{standard deviation}}{\sqrt{N}}$$

$$\text{Standard error} = \frac{10.9}{\sqrt{106}}$$

Standard error $= 1.059$.

$90\% \, CI = \text{Mean} \pm (1.65 \times 1.059) = 61.6 \pm 1.75 = 59.9 \text{ to } 63.3 \text{ micrograms/mL.}$

$95\% \, CI = \text{Mean} \pm (1.96 \times 1.059) = 61.6 \pm 2.08 = 59.5 \text{ to } 63.7 \text{ micrograms/mL.}$

$99\% \, CI = \text{Mean} \pm (2.58 \times 1.059) = 61.6 \pm 2.73 = 58.9 \text{ to } 64.3 \text{ micrograms/mL.}$

---

**EXAMPLE 8:18**

**Question:** You know the mean weight and standard deviation of the population of a tablet batch. You take a sample from this population and calculate the 90% confidence interval for the mean. This interval contains values that are within how many standard errors of the mean?

**Answer:** 1.65.

**EXAMPLE 8:19**

**Question:** The weights of six tablets are measured as: 102.5 mg, 101.7 mg, 103.1 mg, 100.9 mg, 100.5 mg, and 102.2 mg. Calculate the sample mean, standard deviation, and standard error. From this, calculate the confidence interval for the population mean at a 95% confidence level.

**Answer:** First you calculate the mean:

$$\text{Mean} = \frac{x_1 + x_2 + x_3 + \dots + x_n}{n}$$

$$\text{Mean} = \frac{102.5 + 101.7 + 103.1 + 100.9 + 100.5 + 102.2}{6} = 101.8 \text{mg.}$$

$$\text{Standard deviation of a sample} = \sqrt{\frac{\sum (deviation)^2}{N-1}} = 0.985.$$

$$\text{Standard error} = \frac{standard\ deviation}{\sqrt{N}} = 0.402.$$

$$95\% \text{ CI} = \text{Mean} \pm (1.96 \times 0.402) = 101.8 \pm 0.79 = 101.0 - 102.6 \text{ mg.}$$

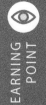

**LEARNING POINT**

## Confidence intervals

Confidence intervals give the probability that a sample of data will contain the true mean. To calculate the confidence intervals for data that conforms to a normal distribution, the following equations are used:

90% confidence interval = mean ± (1.65 × SEM).

95% confidence interval = mean ± (1.96 × SEM).

99% confidence interval = mean ± (2.58 × SEM).

### 8.5.1.1 Using confidence intervals to determine if estimates are significantly different

When considering data it is useful to determine whether or not two estimates are significantly different. When data sets are described as being significantly different, this suggests that it is probable that the difference measured between the data sets is not a result of chance alone. Confidence intervals are a relatively simple way of considering this. If the confidence intervals from two data sets do not overlap, the difference between the sets is significantly different. If the confidence intervals overlap, this suggests the data may not be significantly different. However, formal statistical testing is required to confirm this (see section 8.5.2).

**EXAMPLE 8:20**

**Question:** Consider the following data which show the response rates for a new drug and placebo. Based on the confidence intervals, estimate if the data sets are significantly different.

| Group | % Response rate | 95% CI |
|---|---|---|
| A—received drug | 68.8 | 56.3-79.0 |
| B—placebo | 45.7 | 36.2-55.7 |

**Answer:** In the table, group A shows a higher response rate, but is this significantly higher? By comparing the 95% CI, the confidence intervals do not overlap. Therefore this suggests that the two groups are significantly different, although formal statistical testing is recommended.

**EXAMPLE 8:21**

**Question:** Two groups of patients are attempting to give up smoking; both groups use a nicotine replacement therapy. In addition, group A uses a homeopathic remedy and group B uses a placebo formulation. Consider if the results suggest a significant difference in the results.

| Group | % Response rate | 95% CI |
|---|---|---|
| A—homeopathic | 81.1 | 72.4-87.4 |
| B—placebo | 85.4 | 75.7-91.6 |

**Answer:** In the table, group B shows a higher response rate, but the confidence intervals overlap. Therefore this suggests that the two groups are not significantly different, although formal statistical testing is required.

---

**Confidence intervals and significant difference**

Confidence intervals can be used to indicate if data sets are significantly different.

If the confidence intervals of the two data sets do not overlap, this suggests that the data sets are significantly different.

If the confidence intervals of the two data sets do overlap, the results may not be significantly different, although formal statistical testing is required.

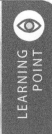

LEARNING POINT

## 8.5.2 Statistical hypothesis testing

Hypothesis testing involves establishing assumptions on the likelihood of an event, and then testing these assumptions. One example could be considering whether blood pressure is different between two groups of people. A second example could be the consideration of manufacture of an antibiotic suspension of a required specification, for example drug content. A batch of 100 bottles removed from production should conform to the product specification for drug content. Therefore the hypothesis is that the specification of the 100 bottles will match that of the product specification. The assumption is that the mean of the sample (in this case the 100 bottles) should be representative of the population mean. This is commonly referred to as the **null hypothesis ($H_0$)**. Basically, the null hypothesis assumes:

- There is no real effect or difference between the measurements from the groups.
  - For example, there is no difference between the blood pressure of the two groups.
- Any difference is a consequence of random errors.

The opposite of a null hypothesis is the **alternative hypothesis ($H_a$)**, which assumes:

- There is a real effect and there is a difference between the measurements from different groups.

We can use a significance test to decide if we should accept or reject the hypothesis. Therefore, we consider this as a measure of how confident we are that the null hypothesis is correct or not. To do this, it is necessary to state the level of confidence or significance under which we accept or reject the null hypothesis. Commonly a significance level of 5% is set.

A p-value is calculated to assess whether the effect seen is likely to have occurred simply through chance, that is there is no real effect and the null hypothesis is true. So the p-value is the probability that we would observe effects as big as those measured in the experiment if there was no difference between the two samples. The p-value selected is arbitrary, but normally it is set as $p < 0.05$. Therefore if the p-value is less than the 5% significance level selected (i.e. $p < 0.05$), this means there is less than a 1 in 20 chance that the difference seen in the data is a result of chance (and you can reject the null hypothesis). Therefore, it is unlikely that the difference in the measured values occurred by chance. If the p-value is larger than 0.05, the observed differences are likely to be a chance finding. If Example 8:20 is considered again, is there a difference in the blood pressures between groups A and B, where group A received a new test drug and group B received a placebo? If the p-value is less than 0.05, then the null hypothesis is rejected (the null hypothesis being that there was no difference in blood pressure between group A and group B). Therefore there is reasonable evidence to support the alternative hypothesis (i.e. there is a significant difference in blood pressures between group A and group B). When data are reported and a significant difference is noted, the p-value should always be reported. However, it is important to remember that just because data sets are shown to be significantly different, this does not mean the difference is important.

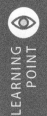

### Statistical significance

Statistically significant does not necessarily mean clinically important. It is the size of the effect that determines the importance, not the presence of statistical significance.

Statistical significance does not necessarily mean the effect is real. Chance also plays a role.

Non-significance does not mean 'no effect'. Small studies will often report non-significance, where a larger study would detect significant differences.

There are a range of statistical tests that can be used to calculate the p-value, and selection of the most appropriate statistical test is dependent on considerations including:

- The type of research question being asked.
- The type of data being analysed.
- The number of groups or data sets involved in the study.

Choosing the right statistical test to compare measurements requires the above factors to be considered. Many statistical tests are based on the assumption that the data are sampled from a Gaussian distribution. These tests are referred to as parametric tests and commonly used parametric tests include the t-test and analysis of variance. Tests that do not make assumptions about the distribution of data are referred to as nonparametric tests. Commonly used nonparametric tests include the Wilcoxon, Mann-Whitney, and Kruskal-Wallis tests. For further details on selecting the most appropriate statistical test, readers are referred to other texts for further development of their statistical understanding[10].

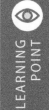

**Statistical significance and p-value.**

A small p-value (typically <0.05) indicates strong evidence against the null hypothesis, meaning it is appropriate to reject it. Therefore if p<0.05, the results compared can be described as significantly different.

A large p-value (>0.05) indicates weak evidence against the null hypothesis, so you cannot reject the null hypothesis (so you cannot reject the conclusion that there is no difference). Therefore the data can be described as not significantly different.

Statistical significance does not necessarily mean the effect is real; if the p-value is 0.05, by chance 1 in 20 significant findings will be spurious.

LEARNING POINT

## 8.6 Self-assessment questions

### 8.6.1 Basic self-assessment questions

This section contains a number of basic self-assessment questions for you to undertake to ensure that you have an understanding of the material in this chapter. It is recommended that you undertake all of these calculations **using a calculator** and then check your answers with the answers in section 8.8.

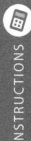

**The use of calculators for the self-assessment questions in this chapter**

It is recommended that you undertake the following calculations using a calculator.

INSTRUCTIONS

10 For example, Jones, D (2002). *Pharmaceutical Statistics*, Pharmaceutical Press, UK.

**QUESTION 8.1:**  *Identify in each of the following experiments what is the independent variable.*

   *a)  You measure the effect of pH on drug solubility.*

   *b)  You measure the drug release from nanoparticles over time.*

   *c)  You measure the amount of digoxin adsorbed onto different masses of carbon black.*

**QUESTION 8.2:**  *The following data show the conversion of degrees Fahrenheit to degrees Celsius:*

| F (°F) | 0 | 50 | 100 | 150 | 200 | 250 |
|--------|-----|-----|------|------|------|-------|
| C (°C) | −17.8 | 10 | 37.8 | 65.6 | 93.9 | 121.1 |

   *a)  From the above data, obtain the equation of the line.*

   *b)  Use the equation of the line to find the Fahrenheit equivalent to 100°C.*

   *c)  Use the equation of the line to find the Celsius equivalent of 98.4°F.*

**QUESTION 8.3:**  *Varying amounts of drug were dissolved in water and the optical absorbance of each solution has been measured. Plot the data and obtain the equation of the line. Use the equation of the line to calculate the drug concentration of a solution that has a UV absorbance of 0.650.*

| Drug concentration (mg/mL) | UV absorption |
|-----------------------------|---------------|
| 0.00 | 0.0 |
| 0.25 | 0.4 |
| 0.50 | 0.8 |
| 0.75 | 1.2 |
| 1.0 | 1.6 |
| 1.5 | 2.3 |

**QUESTION 8.4:**  *The following equations each represent a straight-line plot on a graph. From the equations, identify the gradient and the y-intercept for each.*

   *a)  $y = 6.3x - 10$.*

   *b)  $y = 0.33x$.*

   *c)  $A = ELC_D$ (where A is plotted against $C_D$).*

   *d)  $n/n_0 = 1 + (6.3 \times 10^{21} r^3 C)$ (where $n/n_0$ is plotted against C).*

   *e)  $C/N = C/N_m + 1/(KN_m)$ (where C/N is plotted against C).*

**QUESTION 8.5:**  *Deduce the equation of the straight line, given that the gradient of the line is −3.5 and the line passes through the point (−4,0).*

**QUESTION 8.6:** *Dr W White trains a colleague (J Pinkman) in a drug manufacturing process. Mr Pinkman is able to produce 12 kg of new drug per hour. After 4 hours, the production plant contains 54 kg of new drug. Write an equation to relate the amount of new drug within the building, taking into account the amount Mr Pinkman is producing, assuming no drug is taken from the production site.*

**QUESTION 8.7:** *Two points on the straight-line calibration plot of an absorbance (y) vs concentration (x) graph are:*

- *10 mg/mL, absorbance = 0.3.*
- *50 mg/mL, absorbance = 1.5.*

*Calculate the equation of the line and the concentration equivalent to an absorbance of 0.6.*

**QUESTION 8.8:** *Log linearize the following functions:*

a) $y = 6x^4$.

b) $y = 7x^{-3}$.

c) $C_{tw} = kC_{tt}^2$.

d) $C_{tw} = kC_{tt}^{1/n}$.

**QUESTION 8.9:** *You are presented with the following data, which gives the following graph when plotted. Based on the equation of the line, how could you linearize this plot?*

| Time (h) | Gentamicin conc (mg/L) |
|---|---|
| 1 | 5.7 |
| 2 | 4.2 |
| 3 | 3.1 |
| 4 | 2.3 |
| 6 | 1.2 |

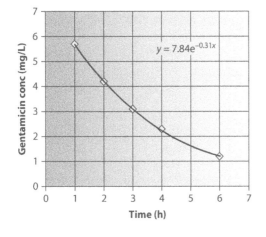

**QUESTION 8.10:** *The pH of a solution of acid varies according to the concentration of solvated protons, [H⁺]:*

| $[H^+] (mol\ dm^{-3})$ | $10^{-1}$ | $10^{-2}$ | $10^{-3}$ | $10^{-4}$ | $10^{-6}$ | $10^{-6}$ | $10^{-7}$ |
|---|---|---|---|---|---|---|---|
| pH | 1 | 2 | 3 | 4 | 5 | 6 | 7 |

*These data fit the following equation: $[H^+] = 10^{-pH}$.*

*Use the data in this table to show we can linearize this equation using natural logarithms.*

**QUESTION 8.11:** *To investigate the stability of a drug in solution, the drug concentration is measured over time. The degradation process is shown to follow zero order kinetics. If the initial drug concentration is 55 mg/mL, what concentration will be remaining after 6 days if the rate constant $k_o = 0.98/day$?*

**QUESTION 8.12:** *A drug is shown to degrade by first order rate kinetics. If the rate constant $k = 0.013/day$, what percentage of drug will remain after 213 days?*

**QUESTION 8.13:** *A drug is shown to degrade by first order rate kinetics. If the rate constant $k_1 = 0.025/day$, what concentration of drug is required to ensure that 60 mg/mL of drug is in solution after 4 days?*

**QUESTION 8.14:** *From the following data, estimate the rate constant of a new drug solution at 25°C. Calculate the shelf-life of the drug solution at 25°C, assuming the degradation of the drug follows first order reaction kinetics where the concentration decreases with time as follows: $\ln C_t = \ln C_0 - k.t$.*

| Temperature (°C) | k (/day) |
|---|---|
| 70 | 0.051 |
| 60 | 0.025 |
| 50 | 0.013 |
| 40 | 0.006 |

**QUESTION 8.15:** *From the following data, estimate the rate constant of a new drug solution at 25°C. Calculate the shelf-life of the drug solution at 25°C, assuming the degradation of the drug follows first order reaction kinetics where the concentration decreases with time as follows: $\ln C_t = \ln C_0 - k.t$.*

| Temperature (°C) | k (/day) |
|---|---|
| 60 | 0.04 |
| 40 | 0.01 |

**QUESTION 8.16:** *The concentration of a drug in the plasma of a group of patients (n = 31) was 127 ± 7 mmol/L (mean ± SD). Calculate the 90%, 95%, and 99% confidence intervals assuming the data originate from a normal distribution.*

**QUESTION 8.17:** *Consider the following results in the comparison of a new drug to reduce blood pressure vs placebo in a study. Use the 95% confidence intervals to consider if the differences seen are significant.*

| | % Number of cases of reduced blood pressure (95% CI) |
|---|---|
| **Group receiving new drug** | 8.5% (7.6–9.1) |
| **Placebo group** | 8.1% (7.2–8.7) |

**QUESTION 8.18:** *Consider the following exam results from two groups of students. From the table, calculate the standard error of the mean and the 95% confidence interval for both groups and consider if the results are significantly different.*

| | Exam results Mean (SD) |
|---|---|
| **Group A (n=110)** | 71.6 (10.9) |
| **Group B (n=127)** | 61.6 (8.5) |

## 8.6.2 Running case studies

**QUESTION 8.19:**

*Marcus has been researching the effectiveness of a new medicine that he thinks could help treat his depression. He came across some clinical data on the internet and has visited your pharmacy to ask about it. The data are below. Looking at the data presented, is there a significant difference between the groups?*

| | % Number of patients reporting a positive outcome (95% CI) |
|---|---|
| **Group receiving drug** | 92% (87–96) |
| **Placebo group** | 68% (62–77) |

**QUESTION 8.20:**

*Marcus also read an article about the positive benefit of homeopathic remedies. He is cynical about such treatments but asks you to interpret the following data for him. How would you interpret these data for Marcus?*

| Group | % Response rate | 95% CI |
|---|---|---|
| **A—homeopathic** | 10.1 | 8.4–11.4 |
| **B—placebo** | 12.4 | 10.2–13.1 |

## 8.7 Summary

A key factor in the stability of medicines is drug degradation. Degradation, like other reaction processes, may follow zero order, first order, pseudo-first order, or second order kinetics. By analysis of stability data we can gain insight into the reaction kinetics involved and the long-term stability and shelf-life of products.

In the analysis of results, data visualization and interpretation is key in forming appropriate conclusions from data sets. In this process it is particularly important to appreciate the application of statistics. Statistics can be used and abused, so a working knowledge of basic statistics is a useful tool; it allows us to compare data sets, make predictions, and draw conclusions from data sets.

## 8.8 Answers to self-assessment questions

This section contains the worked answers for the self-assessment questions within section 8.6.

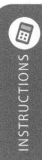

INSTRUCTIONS

### The use of calculators for the self-assessment questions in this chapter

It is recommended that you undertake the following calculations using a calculator.

---

**QUESTION 8.1:**   *Identify in each of the following experiments what is the independent variable.*

*a) You measure the effect of pH on drug solubility.*

*b) You measure the drug release from nanoparticles over time.*

*c) You measure the amount of digoxin adsorbed onto different masses of carbon black.*

**ANSWER:**   a) pH.

b) Time.

c) Carbon black mass.

---

**QUESTION 8.2:**    *The following data show the conversion of degrees Fahrenheit to degrees Celsius:*

| F (°F) | 0 | 50 | 100 | 150 | 200 | 250 |
|--------|------|----|------|------|------|-------|
| C (°C) | −17.8 | 10 | 37.8 | 65.6 | 93.9 | 121.1 |

a) *From the above data, obtain the equation of the line.*

b) *Use the equation of the line to find the Fahrenheit equivalent to 100°C.*

c) *Use the equation of the line to find the Celsius equivalent of 98.4°F.*

**ANSWER:**

a) The equation of the line is: $C = 0.557°F - 17.8$.

b) 100°C is equivalent to 212°F.

c) 98.4°F is equivalent to 37°C.

**QUESTION 8.3:**    *Varying amounts of drug were dissolved in water and the optical absorbance of each solution has been measured. Plot the data and obtain the equation of the line. Use the equation of the line to calculate the drug concentration of a solution that has a UV absorbance of 0.650.*

| Drug concentration (mg/mL) | UV absorption |
|----------------------------|---------------|
| 0.00 | 0.0 |
| 0.25 | 0.4 |
| 0.50 | 0.8 |
| 0.75 | 1.2 |
| 1.0 | 1.6 |
| 1.5 | 2.3 |

**ANSWER:**

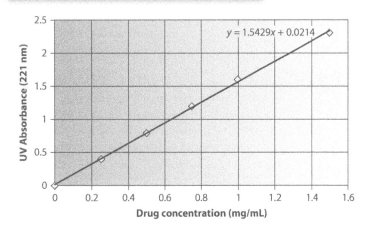

From the graph, we can see the data fit well to a straight-line plot and the equation of the line shows that the intercept is 0.0214 and the gradient is 1.543.

The concentration of a drug solution with a UV absorbance of 0.650 is calculated as follows:

$y =$ UV absorbance of the drug solution $= 0.650$.

$x =$ drug concentration.

Therefore $0.650 = 1.5429x + 0.0214$.

$1.5429\,x = 0.650 - 0.0214$.

$x = 0.41$ mg/mL.

Therefore, the drug concentration of the solution is 0.41 mg/mL.

---

**QUESTION 8.4:** *The following equations each represent a straight-line plot on a graph. From the equations, identify the gradient and the y-intercept for each.*

    *a) $y = 6.3x - 10$.*

    *b) $y = 0.33x$.*

    *c) $A = ELC_D$ (where A is plotted against $C_D$).*

    *d) $n/n_0 = 1 + 6.3 \times 10^{21} r^3 C$ (where $n/n_0$ is plotted against C).*

    *e) $C/N = C/N_m + 1/(KN_m)$ (where C/N is plotted against C).*

**ANSWER:**     a) Gradient is 6.3, y-intercept is $-10$.

    b) Gradient is 0.33, y-intercept is 0.

    c) Gradient is EL, y-intercept is 0.

    d) Gradient is $6.3 \times 10^{21} r^3$, y-intercept is 1.

    e) Gradient is $1/N_m$, and y-intercept is $1/(KN_m)$.

---

**QUESTION 8.5:** *Deduce the equation of the straight line, given that the gradient of the line is $-3.5$ and the line passes through the point $(-4,0)$.*

**ANSWER:** The equation of the line is: $y = mx + c$ and $m = -3.5$.

Therefore: $y = -3.5x + c$; however, we still need to calculate $c$, and we know when $x = -4$, $y = 0$.

$0 = (-3.5 \times (-4)) + c$, and thus $c = -14$.

Therefore the equation of the line is $y = -3.5x - 14$.

---

**QUESTION 8.6:** *Dr W White trains a colleague (J Pinkman) in a drug manufacturing process. Mr Pinkman is able to produce 12 kg of new drug per hour. After 4 hours, the production plant contains 54 kg of new drug. Write an equation to relate the amount of new drug within the building, taking into account the amount Mr Pinkman is producing, assuming no drug is taken from the production site.*

**ANSWER:** The equation of the line is: $y = mx + c$ and $m = 12$ kg per hour.

Therefore: $y = 12x + c$; however, we still need to calculate $c$.

In the above example, after 4 hours, 48 kg of drug is produced and we have a total of 54 kg of new drug in the production plant, so:

$54 = 48 + c$, and thus $c = 6$.

Therefore the equation of the line is $y = 12x + 6$.

**QUESTION 8.7:**  Two points on the straight-line calibration plot of an absorbance (y) vs concentration (x) graph are:

- 10 mg/mL, absorbance = 0.3.
- 50 mg/mL, absorbance = 1.5.

Calculate the equation of the line and the concentration equivalent to an absorbance of 0.6.

**ANSWER:**

$$m = \frac{change\ in\ y}{change\ in\ x} = \frac{y_2 - y_1}{x_2 - x_1} = \frac{\Delta y}{\Delta x}$$

$$= (1.5-0.3)/(50-10)$$

$$= 0.03$$

The equation of the line is: $y = mx + c$ and $m = 0.03$.

Therefore, $y = 0.03x + c$; however, we still need to calculate $c$.

You can use either of the two points for $x$ and $y$:

$$c = 0.3 - (0.03 \times 10)$$

$c = 0$, and the equation of the line is $y = 0.03x$

To calculate the concentration equivalent to an absorbance of 0.6:

$$y = 0.03x$$

Therefore, $0.6 = 0.03x$.

$$x = 20\ mg/mL.$$

**QUESTION 8.8:**  Log linearize the following functions:

a) $y = 6x^4$.

b) $y = 7x^{-3}$.

c) $C_{tw} = kC_{tt}^2$.

d) $C_{tw} = kC_{tt}^{1/n}$.

**ANSWER:**

a) $log(y) = 0.78 + 4log(x)$.

b) $log(y) = 0.85 - 3log(x)$.

c) $log(C_{tw}) = log(k) + 2log(C_{tt})$.

d) $log(C_{tw}) = log(k) + (1/n)log(C_{tt})$.

**QUESTION 8.9:**  You are presented with the following data, which gives the following graph when plotted. Based on the equation of the line, how could you linearize this plot?

| Time (h) | Gentamicin conc (mg/L) |
|---|---|
| 1 | 5.7 |
| 2 | 4.2 |
| 3 | 3.1 |
| 4 | 2.3 |
| 6 | 1.2 |

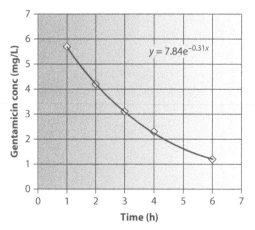

**ANSWER:** The equation is in the general format of $y = km^x$, plotting $log(y)$ on the y-axis and $x$ on the x-axis, will give you a straight-line plot where $log(m)$ is the gradient and $log(k)$ is the intercept. Given that $m = e$, natural logs can be used.

Natural log linearization of the equation:

$y = 7.84e^{-0.31x}$.

$ln(y) = ln(7.84) - 0.31x ln(e)$.

$ln(y) = 2.06 - 0.31x$  (remember $ln(e) = 1$).

**QUESTION 8.10:** The pH of a solution of acid varies according to the concentration of solvated protons, $[H^+]$:

| $[H^+]$ (mol dm$^{-3}$) | $10^{-1}$ | $10^{-2}$ | $10^{-3}$ | $10^{-4}$ | $10^{-6}$ | $10^{-6}$ | $10^{-7}$ |
|---|---|---|---|---|---|---|---|
| pH | 1 | 2 | 3 | 4 | 5 | 6 | 7 |

These data fit the following equation: $[H^+] = 10^{-pH}$.

Use the data in this table to show we can linearize this equation using natural logarithms.

**ANSWER:** Either ln or log can be used here. For example:

$ln[H^+] = ln(10^{-pH})$.

$ln[H^+] = -pH\ ln(10)$.

$ln[H^+] = -2.303\ pH$.

Therefore if we now plot the graph of $ln[H+]$ on the y-axis against pH, we should get a straight line with a gradient of $-2.303$, and an intercept $= 0$, as shown below.

| $[H^+]$/mol dm$^{-3}$ | $10^{-1}$ | $10^{-2}$ | $10^{-3}$ | $10^{-4}$ | $10^{-6}$ | $10^{-6}$ | $10^{-7}$ |
|---|---|---|---|---|---|---|---|
| ln $[H^+]$ | -2.303 | -4.605 | -6.908 | -9.21 | -11.53 | -13.82 | -16.18 |
| pH | 1 | 2 | 3 | 4 | 5 | 6 | 7 |

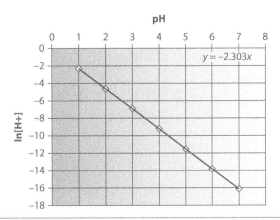

**QUESTION 8.11:** *To investigate the stability of a drug in solution the drug concentration is measured over time. The degradation process is shown to follow zero order kinetics. If the initial drug concentration is 55 mg/mL, what concentration will remain after 6 days if the rate constant $k_0 = 0.98$/day?*

**ANSWER:**
$C_t = C_0 - k_0 t.$

$C_t = 55\,\text{mg/mL} - (0.98 \times 6).$

$C_t = 49.12\,\text{mg/mL}.$

**QUESTION 8.12:** A drug is shown to degrade by first order rate kinetics. If the rate constant $k = 0.013$/day, what percentage of drug will remain after 213 days?

**ANSWER:**
$\ln C_t = \ln C_0 - k.t.$

$\ln C_t = \ln 100 - 0.013 \times 213.$

$\ln C_t = 4.61 - 2.77 = 1.84.$

$C_t = 6.3\%$, therefore 6.3% of the drug will be remaining after 213 days.

**QUESTION 8.13:** *A drug is shown to degrade by first order rate kinetics. If the rate constant $k_1 = 0.025$/day, what concentration of drug is required to ensure that 60 mg/mL of drug is in solution after 4 days?*

**ANSWER:**
We know we want $C_t = 60\,\text{mg/mL}$ after 4 days, so we need to identify what the starting concentration ($C_0$) should be.

$\ln C_t = \ln C_0 - k.t.$

$\ln 60 = \ln C_0 - (0.025 \times 4).$

$\ln 60 = \ln C_0 - 0.1.$

$\ln C_0 = 4.09 + 0.1 = 4.19.$

$C_0 = 66\,\text{mg/mL}.$

**QUESTION 8.14:** *From the following data, estimate the rate constant of a new drug solution at 25°C. Calculate the shelf-life of the drug solution at 25°C, assuming the degradation of the drug follows first order reaction kinetics where the concentration decreases with time as follows:*
$\ln C_t = \ln C_0 - k.t.$

| Temperature (°C) | k (/day) |
|---|---|
| 70 | 0.051 |
| 60 | 0.025 |
| 50 | 0.013 |
| 40 | 0.006 |

ANSWER: First we need to calculate 1/T (in Kelvin) and ln k.

| Temperature (°C) | k (/day) | T(K) | 1/T | ln k |
|---|---|---|---|---|
| 70 | 0.051 | 343 | 0.0029 | −2.98 |
| 60 | 0.025 | 333 | 0.0030 | −3.69 |
| 50 | 0.013 | 323 | 0.0031 | −4.34 |
| 40 | 0.006 | 313 | 0.0032 | −5.12 |

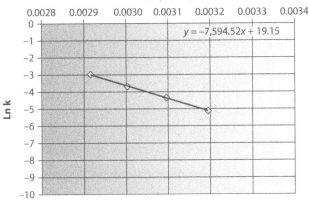

From this we can now calculate k at 25°C (298K):

ln k = 19.15 − 7594.52/T.

ln k = 19.15 − 25.48 = −6.33.

Therefore k = 0.0017 (this can also be done by extrapolation of the line).

At a shelf-life of 90% of the stated active ingredient remaining:

$C_t = C_0.e^{-kt}$, where $C_t$ = drug concentration at 90%, $C_0$ is 100%, and k we have calculated at 25°C. Therefore:

$\ln C_t = \ln C_0 - k.t$.

$$t = \frac{\ln(\frac{C_0}{C_t})}{k} = \frac{\ln(\frac{100}{90})}{0.0017} = 62 \text{ days}.$$

Therefore the shelf-life of the product is 62 days at 25°C.

**QUESTION 8.15:** *From the following data, estimate the rate constant of a new drug solution at 25°C. Calculate the shelf-life of the drug solution at 25°C, assuming the degradation of the drug follows first order reaction kinetics where the concentration decreases with time as follows: $\ln C_t = \ln C_0 - k.t$.*

| Temperature (°C) | k (/day) |
|---|---|
| 60 | 0.04 |
| 40 | 0.01 |

**ANSWER:** First we need to calculate 1/T (in Kelvin) and ln k.

| Temperature (°C) | k (day⁻¹) | T(K) | 1/T | ln k |
|---|---|---|---|---|
| 60 | 0.04 | 333 | 0.0030 | −3.22 |
| 40 | 0.01 | 313 | 0.0032 | −4.61 |

The gradient is calculated as:

$$m = \frac{change\ in\ y}{change\ in\ x} = \frac{y_2 - y_1}{x_2 - x_1} = \frac{\Delta y}{\Delta x}$$

$$= (-3.22 - (-4.61)) \div (0.0030 - 0.0032).$$

$$= 1.39 \div (-0.0002) = -6950.$$

The equation of the line is: $y = mx + c$ and $m = -6950$, therefore:

$$-3.22 = (-6950 * 0.0030) + c$$

$$c = 17.63.$$

From this we can now calculate k at 25°C (298K):

$$\ln k = 17.63 - 6950/T.$$

$$\ln k = 17.63 - 23.32 = -5.69.$$

Therefore k = 0.0034.

At a shelf-life of 90% of the stated active ingredient remaining:

$C_t = C_0.e^{-kt}$, where $C_t$ = drug concentration at 90%, $C_0$ is 100%, and k we have calculated at 25°C. Therefore:

$$\ln C_t = \ln C_0 - k.t.$$

$$t = \frac{\ln(\frac{C_0}{C_t})}{k} = \frac{\ln(\frac{100}{90})}{0.0034} = 31\ days.$$

Therefore the shelf-life of the product is 31 days at 25°C.

**QUESTION 8.16:** *The concentration of a drug in the plasma of a group of patients (n = 31) was 127 ± 7 mmol/L (mean ± SD). Calculate the 90%, 95%, and 99% confidence intervals assuming the data originate from a normal distribution.*

**ANSWER:** First you calculate the standard error of the mean:

$$\text{Standard error} = \frac{\textit{standard deviation}}{\sqrt{N}}$$

$$\text{Standard error} = \frac{7}{\sqrt{31}}$$

Standard error = 1.26.

90% CI = mean ± (1.65 × 1.26) = 127 ± (2.07) = 125 to 129 mmol/L.

95% CI = mean ± (1.96 × 1.26) = 127 ± (2.46) = 125 to 130 mmol/L.

99% CI = mean ± (2.58 × 1.26) = 127 ± (3.24) = 124 to 130 mmol/L.

**QUESTION 8.17:** *Consider the following results in the comparison of a new drug to reduce blood pressure vs placebo in a study. Use the 95% confidence intervals to consider if the differences seen are significant.*

|  | % Number of cases of reduced blood pressure (95% CI) |
|---|---|
| **Group receiving new drug** | 8.5% (7.6−9.1) |
| **Placebo group** | 8.1% (7.2−8.7) |

**ANSWER:** In this study the confidence intervals overlap, therefore it cannot be confirmed that the values are statistically different and additional statistical testing to find the p-value should be considered.

**QUESTION 8.18:** *Consider the following exam results from two groups of students. From the table, calculate the standard error of the mean and the 95% confidence interval for both groups and consider if the results are significantly different.*

|  | Exam results Mean (SD) |
|---|---|
| **Group A (n = 110)** | 71.6 (10.9) |
| **Group B (n = 127)** | 61.6 (8.5) |

**ANSWER:**

$$\text{Group A standard error} = \frac{\textit{standard deviation}}{\sqrt{N}}$$

$$\text{Group A standard error} = \frac{10.9}{\sqrt{110}}$$

Standard error = 1.039.

Group A 95% CI = Mean ± (1.96 × 1.039) = 71.6 ± (2.04) = 69.6 to 73.6%.

$$\text{Group B standard error} = \frac{8.5}{\sqrt{127}}$$

Standard error = 0.75.

$95\% \, CI = 61.6 \pm (1.96 \times 0.75) = 61.6 \pm 1.47 = 60.1 \, to \, 63.1\%.$

In this study the confidence intervals do not overlap suggesting these results are significantly different.

---

**QUESTION 8.19:**

*Marcus has been researching the effectiveness of a new medicine that he thinks could help treat his depression. He came across some clinical data on the internet and has visited your pharmacy to ask about it. The data are below. Looking at the data presented, is there a significant difference between the groups?*

| | % Number of patients reporting a positive outcome (95% CI) |
|---|---|
| **Group receiving drug** | 92% (87 – 96) |
| **Placebo group** | 68% (62 – 77) |

**ANSWER:**

In this study the confidence intervals do not overlap, suggesting these results are significantly different.

---

**QUESTION 8.20:**

*Marcus also read an article about the positive benefit of homeopathic remedies. He is cynical about such treatments but asks you to interpret the following data for him. How would you interpret this data for Marcus?*

| Group | % Response rate | 95% CI |
|---|---|---|
| **A—homeopathic** | 10.1 | 8.4 – 11.4 |
| **B—placebo** | 12.4 | 10.2 – 13.1 |

**ANSWER:**

In this study the confidence intervals overlap, suggesting there is no significant difference in the results and therefore Marcus should not waste his money on homeopathic remedies. In general, there is no clinical evidence to support the effectiveness of any homeopathic remedy beyond the placebo effect; however, the sugar used in some formulations can cause dental cavities.

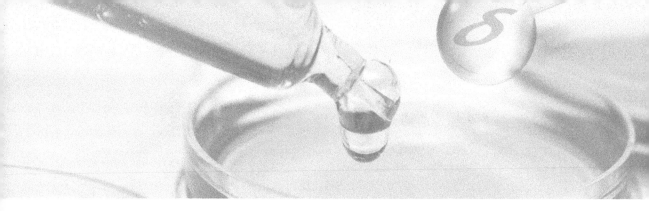

# Appendix: Pharmaceutical administration abbreviations

| | |
|---|---|
| aa (ana) | of each |
| ac (ante cibum) | before food |
| ad/add (addendus) | to be added (up to) |
| ad lib (ad libitum) | as much as desired |
| alt (alternus) | alternate |
| alt die (alterno die) | every other day |
| applic (applicetur) | let it be applied |
| bd/bid (bis die/bis in die) | twice a day |
| c (cum) | with |
| cc (cum cibus) | with food |
| corp (corpori) | to the body |
| d (dies) | a day |
| dd (de die) | daily |
| dil (dilutes) | diluted |
| div (divide) | divide |
| et (et) | and |
| ex aq (ex aqua) | in water |
| freq (frequenter) | frequently |
| h (hora) | at the hour |
| hs (hora somni) | at the hour of sleep (bedtime) |
| ic (inter cibos) | between meals |
| m/mane (mane) | in the morning |
| md (more dicto) | as directed |
| mdu (more dicto utendus) | use as directed |
| mitt/mitte (mitte) | send (quantity to be given) |
| n/nocte (nocte) | at night |
| n et m (nocte maneque) | night and morning |
| ocul (oculo) | to (for) the eye |
| od (omni die) | every day |
| oh (omni hora) | every hour |
| om (omni mane) | every morning |
| on (omni nocte) | every night |
| paa (parti affectae applicandus) | apply to the affected part |
| pc (post cibum) | after food |
| po (per os) | by mouth |
| pr (per rectum) | rectally |
| prn (pro re nata) | when required |
| pv (per vagina) | vaginally |
| qds/qid (quater die sumendum/quater in die) | four times a day |
| qqh/q4h (quarta quaque hora) | every 4 hours |
| qs (quantum sufficiat) | sufficient |
| R (recipe) | take |
| solv (solve) | dissolve |
| sos (si opus sit) | when necessary |
| stat (statim) | immediately |
| tds/tid (ter die sumendum/ter in die) | three times a day |
| tuss urg (tussi urgente) | when the cough is troublesome |
| ut dict/ud (ut dictum) | as directed |

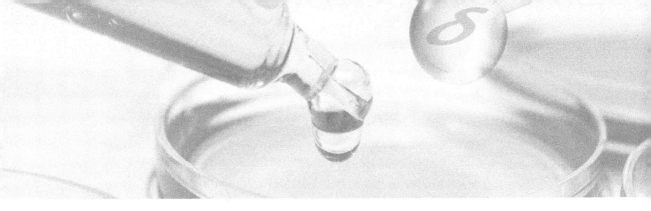

# Index